When Your Friend Gets
CANCER

How you can help

by Amy Harwell
with Kristine Tomasik

Harold Shaw Publishers
Wheaton, Illinois

Christina
Thank you for
making these
books available
to your community
I'm hopeful they
witness love.
Amy 10·15·88
Blessings to you &
your father, too.

Cover photo © George A. Robinson

ISBN 0–87788–934–1

Library of Congress Cataloging-in-Publication Data
Harwell, Amy.
    When your friend gets cancer.

    Bibliography: p.
    Includes index.
    1. Cancer—Psychological aspects.   2. Helping behavior.
I. Tomasik, Kristine.   I. Title.
RC262.H34   1987   158'.2   87–9547
ISBN 0–87788–934–1

96 95 94 93 92 91 90 89 88 87

10 9 8 7 6 5 4 3 2

To Polly,
my "angel on earth"
and
Jayne and Jess,
my parents,
who proved family
can be friends

Contents

Contents

Foreword

Amy Harwell. The name sounded familiar. Though I was fairly new at St. Mark's Episcopal Church in Geneva, Illinois, I remembered hearing it voiced regularly during the intercessory prayers on Sunday mornings, when people in the congregation lift their friends and loved ones to God by name for his help.

And I had heard church friends fondly mention Amy Harwell in conversation. I learned that she was a former parishioner of St. Mark's, now living and working in Chicago. One day someone announced to me, with obvious excitement, "Amy's speaking on cancer to the Adult Discussion Group next Sunday."

"What qualifies her to give a talk about cancer?" I wondered aloud. (My husband had died of cancer less than a year before, and I had a much-more-than-casual interest in the subject.)

"She has it," was the reply.

Well, O.K. So someone who had terminal cancer was willing to talk about it to a church group. That would take some chutzpah, I admitted. But I knew from experience that a lay-person's presentation might well be morbid, ill-informed, sentimental, self-centered, garbled, or a spiel for some off-the-wall cancer treatment. Curious, I knew I would be there to find out.

The group in the choir room was larger than usual that Sunday morning. As I entered I felt the air charged with anticipation. And there, enfolded in a knot of enthusiastically hugging humans, stood Amy. A glance at her dispelled one fear. She certainly didn't look like someone with cancer.

Not only was Amy there, chic, dark-haired, bright-eyed, bubbly, vivacious, charming, but surrounding her chair was a large collection of miscellaneous objects (why did she bring all her household goods with her?), and standing next to her was a flip chart, complete with colored felt markers.

As she began to talk I remember being spell-bound, drawn into her warm and fluent telling of her own story, punctuated with fear-words like "bleeding," and "hospital," and "tests," and "tumors," and "doctors," and "chemotherapy," but also with hope-words—"friends," and "flowers," and "loving," and "God," and surprisingly, "healing."

And Amy wasn't necessarily talking about physical healing. Apart from a slight huskiness and cough, she seemed robust enough, but what was remarkable was her air of confidence, of emotional wholeness and energy, of spiritual vitality. For an hour the choir room was filled with show-and-tell (that's what the teddy-bears, and photographs, and books, and baskets of gifts and cards were all about), questions and answers, authoritative statistics and colorful diagrams and lists that were far from the merely academic. They broadened the discussion from one cancer patient's personal, anecdotal history to include each of us, to acquaint us with the facts, to tell us our own chances, and to show us how we could be Jesus-friends to someone with cancer.

For me, much of what she said was like walking again through familiar, rocky territory. As the survivor of a spouse who died of lung cancer, I could nod my head with tears in my eyes and affirm, "Yes. That's what we learned; that's what it's like; that's what we had to go through. I've felt those ups and downs. And I know how important strong, loving friends are when someone you love has cancer." What impressed me was how clearly Amy had thought through the stages of cancer, the interlocking of the physical, spiritual, and emotional processes and pain, her insights into how they all work together, how you can live with them. How you must be prepared also to die with them. But to die whole.

"This woman is a born communicator," I thought to myself. "Not only so, but she's a thinker. She's developed a philosophy of cancer and friendship, and a living theology that is far from stoic or fatalistic." Though she herself had been given a very negative prognosis, somehow, instead of disillusionment and despair, she had found hope and meaning, and exercised her considerable skills to help the rest of us see the gleams in the dark landscape through her eyes.

After the hour was over, I couldn't help myself—I went over to Amy, hugged her, and said, "You must put all of this in a book. And I'll publish it." She looked incredulous. Then apprehensive.

But she got over it. She wrote the book, putting her whole self into it. And we've published it.

Now, it's up to you to read it. And act on it.

Luci Shaw

Dear Reader

You just found out. Your friend has cancer.

You're shocked. "Oh, no—not her!" You're disbelieving. "It can't be—she's so vital!" And perhaps, most of all, you're overwhelmed. "What can I ever do to help her?"

This welter of feelings is normal. Denial, grief, numbness, confusion, anxiety, even anger are all reactions we have to crushing news about someone we hold dear.

But one thing I beg of you: don't let your emotions paralyze you. Reach out to your friend now—no matter how inadequate you feel. She needs all the affirmation she can get, no matter how small your comfort may seem to you in the face of her giant crisis. Your gift is not small. You are a very significant person. You are a friend. Friends come in all shapes and sizes—acquaintances, neighbors, coworkers, fellow church members, pals, best friends.

(Note to the reader: I chose the pronoun "she" because most book readers are "she's," and most friends are same-sex. For ease of reading I'll retain this style, but am confident that all that follows is pertinent to female/male and male friendships as well.)

Though not a substitute for family, friends hold a special niche in the life of a cancer patient. Because they are not as close as family, friends can listen to fears more readily. Because they are not as dependent on the patient, friends can be less frightened about the consequences of treatment and can usually live better in the ambiguity of the situation. Friends can objectively help the cancer patient get through the cancer crisis.

How do I know all this?

In July of 1985 I, a single career woman, 35 years old, was diagnosed as having invasive cervical cancer, with an eighty percent recovery prognosis. When subsequent biopsies and surgery revealed significant lymph node involvement, my prognosis dropped to fifty percent. When more nodes tested malignant, it dropped to thirty percent. Not satisfied with leaving things in statistical terms, I asked my physician, "Who in your personal experience has lived to the five-year mark with my type and spread of cancer?"

"No one," he replied.

Treatment was extensive—ten weeks in the hospital, spread over a total of five months. During my cancer crisis I underwent four trips to the operating table, fifty radiation treatments, a radiation implant, and thirty days of twenty-four-hour-a-day intravenous chemotherapy.

Without the loving help, support, and reassurance of my friends, I don't know what I would have done. They sent me cards and flowers, they called me, they ran errands, they prayed. I'm writing this book for two reasons: as a big thank-you to all of them, and to let you in on the combined richness of their wisdom and the practicality of their gifts.

From my friends, you can learn the answer to your question, "What can I do?" You can, as they did, follow the seven simple suggestions outlined in this book:

1. *Check your attitudes about cancer and about friendship.* Do you secretly think of cancer as punishment? Does it sound an immediate death-knell in your mind? Then you need to clarify your thinking, because the cancer patient doesn't need people who will judge her and work through their attitudes in front of her now. Also think about the meaning of your friendship.

2. *Reach out immediately and boldly.* The cancer patient is experiencing isolation and alienation. She needs your phone call or card now!

3. *Get prepped on cancer facts, figures, and feelings.* Do some homework to understand basic cancer jargon and the emotional impact of the disease, especially as related to your friend's specific case. She might not have the energy to educate you herself.

4. *Offer your helping hands.* Uplift the cancer patient, encourage her, make her environment more pleasant, do practical nuts-and-bolts chores, support her loved ones, and steer her to other available resources. You have something special to give her that only you can provide.

5. *Share your healing heart.* Listen to the cancer patient. Ask her gently probing questions as she goes through her process of adjustment, especially as she deals with her changing expectations for the future. Embrace her; she needs your physical touch of love. Pray for her.

6. *Help your friend make death and dying decisions (if asked).* Your friend will face major decisions if her prognosis is poor. Help her as she deals with health care ethics, as she explores her relationship with God, and as she deals with her pending death.

7. *Be there for your friend.* Once she has been diagnosed with cancer, her life will never be quite the same. hang in there with her as she lives with the post-treatment blues and faces a new future.

Of course, you will have your own feelings as you watch your friend go through her cancer crisis. Yet your invitation to go through it with her at whatever level of involvement you feel capable of will make it another deeper experience of your friendship. It will not be easy, but your relationship will be the richer for it. In fact, I no longer despair when I hear that someone has cancer. I know what a fertile soil it has been for me to experience profound love, to bond friendships, to find meaning in life, and to appreciate my own God-given talents and abilities.

I know that my cancer has cemented my relationship with God. I have now experienced God the Father as Provider, God the Spirit as Comforter, and God the Son, Jesus, not only as Savior but also as the ultimate and supreme Friend. What a friend I have in Him.

As I give this book into your hands, I'm very aware of the

risk of generalizing from my one set of specific experiences. I trust that you will not do this, but will instead use this book as one example—a foil if you will—to share with your friend as you ferret out necessary facts and feelings together. Use it please.

Sincerely,
Amy

1
Checking Your Attitudes about Cancer and about Friendship

Cancer. Perhaps no other word in the English language is so loaded. When we hear "cancer," immediate knee-jerk associations fill our minds. "Pain," we think. "Suffering." "Nausea." And, perhaps most of all, we think "death." Because these thoughts are so unpleasant, we quickly turn away from them. In so doing, we often unwittingly turn away from the friend who has the cancer. If you are going to help your friend, you need to look at your feelings about cancer. You need to face your own fears and dreads and sort the true from the false, the realistic from the superstitious. Then you will be able to turn toward your friend and be with her.

The Common Cancer
Close to one million people will be diagnosed with cancer this year in the United States (carcinoma in situ and non-melanoma skin cancers are not included). Close to half of a million people

in this country will die of cancer this year—one every seventy seconds. But—good news—there are over three million people living today who have fought cancer and won. These statistics are so staggering it may be hard to get your mind around them. So imagine it this way. Let's say that in 1986 you lived in a small town of 10,000 people. In their booklet "1986 Cancer Facts & Figures," the *American Cancer Society* estimated that in your small community there were thirty-three new cancer cases diagnosed this year and that eighteen people will have died of cancer this year. Of the 10,000 people in your town, 2800 will eventually develop cancer, and 1800 will die of cancer if the present rate continues. To bring it even closer to home, one person in four will be diagnosed with cancer sometime during his or her lifetime. Over the years, cancer will invade approximately three out of four families.

What Is Cancer?
Cancer is a generic term for a large group of diseases. However, most of us don't think "disease" when we hear the word "cancer." We think "dying."

But the *American Cancer Society's* 1986 research reveals that fifty percent of those diagnosed with one of the forms of cancer this year will be alive five years after diagnosis. Other misunderstandings surround this volatile word. One common paranoia about cancer is that it's contagious. The fact is, cancer is not contagious. You cannot catch it by being with someone who has it.

Cancer is a negative word in our popular language, too. We hear of the "cancer of Communism" or how "poverty is spreading like a cancer."

According to the *American Cancer Society*, cancer is a condition of uncontrolled growth and spread of abnormal cells. But medical science still does not know exactly what causes certain cells to go berserk in certain human bodies. And as always, we tend to fear what we do not fully understand.

Why Cancer?

When a friend or loved one is diagnosed as having cancer, one of the first questions we ask is "Why?"

Millions of dollars have been spent researching the following as possible causes of cancer: carcinogens, such as pollution, X-rays, and cigarette smoke; foods, such as red meat or fats; stress, brought on by worry, depression, or loss; genetics; and viruses. According to writers Marion Morra and Eve Potts in their recent and comprehensive handbook on cancer treatment, *Choices*, "Most cancer researchers believe that somehow, usually over a period of years, cancer-causing agents (carcinogens) repeatedly brought into the body finally damage a critical piece of a cell's genetic code. The damage causes the cell to send out abnormal messages related to some aspect of cell growth."

When asked about the cause of cancer, many doctors will simply and honestly say, "Ultimately, we don't know." But no answer about the physiological cause of cancer satisfies the question of why people have to suffer with cancer.

Unfortunately, since cancer can be such a fearsome thing, the human mind is quick to conclude that cancer is punishment. "Cancer is bad, therefore she must have been bad," is the way this thinking goes. Obviously, such thinking is childish—elementary—and just plain wrong. But there's still plenty of it around. At a theological seminar I attended about health care ethics, a clergy member declared, "Clearly, cancer victims are out of grace with God."

We need to weed out such erroneous notions before we see our friend. Bad things do not just happen to "bad" people. Bad things happen to good people. That is the hard and mysterious nature of the universe.

I have heard Christians propose another theory. "Oh, God is going to show his glory through your cancer," they say. In other words, God gave you cancer so he can heal you and thus show his power. That may be a possibility.

But I prefer to think that the "reason" for my cancer experience is for my own personal spiritual refinement. Not long after my cancer struck, my mother asked me, "Amy, do you know how they make steel?"

"No," I said.

She looked me right in the eye and said, "They put it in the fire . . . to make it tougher."

My cancer has had exactly this effect on me; as I went through the fires of radiation and chemotherapy, I perceived it as a refining process God could use to make me better. But better for what?

In his book *Why Not?: Accept Christ's Healing and Wholeness*, Lloyd J. Olgivie suggests an answer. He believes that God keeps on refining us until he can see his own reflection in us.

Like the steel, God's refining process has caused me to shed some of my impurities. To give up the pride. To let go of the control. I hope the net result is that others can better see his reflection in me. What a gift when they do!

How Have You Dealt with Previous Losses?

Your friend's cancer crisis does not arrive in a vacuum. Rather, it comes into your life—a life in which you have experienced previous losses, possibly many from cancer. How healed or unhealed you are from these losses will affect the way you deal with this current threat of loss.

One friend almost completely withdrew from me when she heard of my cancer diagnosis. She told me in no uncertain terms, "Amy, I have nothing to give you emotionally." The reason? Her mother had died of cancer less than a year before. My friend simply had not recovered enough from the open wound of this loss to be able to help me.

Another friend's reaction was exactly the opposite. She had experienced the loss of her father from cancer only a short time previously. But precisely because she felt she had not handled that loss well, she was eager to help me in my crisis. "Amy," she told me firmly, "don't deny me the opportunity of helping you." Helping me was a way of making up for what she hadn't been able to do for her father.

Most friends will probably be able to strike a middle ground. "Yes, I've had previous losses. And despite the reminder of past pain, I will help you."

How Close a Friend Are You?

Friendship definitely has its own life cycle. A relationship is not a static thing, but is constantly in flux.

Some friendships are just beginning. If that is true, the friend will not be as deeply affected by the news of the diagnosis, because she is not as deeply involved.

Some friendships are at the height of reciprocal reward

and therefore will be assaulted the most fiercely by the news of cancer. The friendship has lost its presumed safety. These friends will tend both to give more deeply and to grieve more deeply.

In a waning friendship, other feelings are evoked by the news of the illness. Guilt or sadness over the friendship's coming to a close may make it harder for this person to show much overt caring.

Everyone's definition of friendship is different. Letty Cottin Pogrebin, in her recent book *Among Friends,* gives this one: "Friendship is a heart-flooding feeling that can happen to any two people who are caught up in the act of being themselves, together, and who like what they see."

Pogrebin offers the following "litmus test" of friendship. Friendship, she says, will be characterized by four qualities: acceptance—not a blind adoration, but constructive support; generosity—the practical giving of one's time, effort, or money; honesty—sincerity, which is freedom from deceit; and loyalty and trust—the ability to keep confidences.

Family members also can be friends, as my father reminded me when he sent the book *A Friend Is Someone Special.* The note on the flyleaf read, "Dear Amy, in addition to being your parents, we hope we are your friends."

My favorite definition of friendship continues to be this one by Frances Farmer. She says, "To have a good friend is the purest of all God's gifts, for it is a love that has no exchange of payment. It is not inherited as with a family. It is not compelling as with a child. And it has no means of physical pleasure, as with a mate. It is, therefore, an indescribable bond that brings with it a far deeper devotion than all the others." How true my friends were to this quote!

As you consider how to help the cancer patient, ask yourself seriously, "How close a friend am I?"

What Are You Able—and Willing—to Give?

When your friend gets cancer, it is easy to be overwhelmed at the thought of helping her. You imagine running back and forth to the hospital. You think of the hours you'll be there with her. You may even dread the drain on your precious energy, strength, and endurance. You may fear you will be taxed beyond your limits.

All these are real considerations. That is why you need to think now about how much you are willing to give. That is why you need to know that it is OK to set limits. That is why you need to know it's OK to take time out for yourself.

Here's the vital piece of information. You don't have to do it all by yourself. Through my cancer crisis, I saw that God had set a cosmic care plan into effect for me. Many friends ministered to me in many different ways. Each person did what was unique to him or her. Some played more significant roles than others, but no one person did it all. Together, all these people and their many gifts formed a huge net of support.

So take heart. Measure the scope of your present giving potential, then make your unique contribution. You are part of the Plan.

2
Reaching Out Immediately and Boldly

If you heard that a friend had broken a leg and was in traction in the hospital, what would you do?

You'd probably pick the phone right up and give a jingle. "I just heard about your leg. I'm really sorry! What can I do for you?" Then you'd run out and pop a card in the mail or you might send flowers.

When a friend has cancer you should do *exactly the same things*. In one way, cancer is just a disease—a hurt—a break—like any other illness. Of course, in another way, cancer is not just some other illness. It's cancer, and as soon as we hear it, we all start acting strange. "I was afraid to send you flowers," is a frequent comment. "I was afraid you'd think they were for your funeral."

The fact is, the cancer patient needs your concern all the more—and all the more immediately—precisely because of the diagnosis of cancer. In some ways, the need for treatment isn't as urgent as the cancer patient's need for support. She is caught in "flight or fight" thinking. Will you approach—or avoid?

When a person is diagnosed with cancer, she is tossed immediately into the ring with four large-scale issues. According to the U.S. Department of Health and Human Services and their book *Coping with Cancer,* these are: alienation, loss of control, mutilation, and fear of mortality.

The cancer patient feels *alienation* because she has the big "IT," the big "C." She feels lonely and isolated, cut off from family, neighbors, and friends; errands and to-do lists; work schedules and business opportunities. Instead, she is plunged into a world of steel machines, plastic tubes, and endless white.

The second issue your friend faces is *loss of control.* Clearly her body has betrayed her. She feels very vulnerable. She is no longer sure what is happening to her or how to plan her life. She cannot just assume the future—that what she wants to take place will take place. Everything is up in the air, both short-term and long-term.

Your friend fears *"mutilation"*—also known as an "altered body image." She knows her treatment could easily mean disfiguring surgery. Radiation and chemotherapy have many known and unknown long-term side effects. She has heard more horror stories about these than mere loss of hair, and she wonders what effect her changed body will have on her friends and loved ones.

The cancer patient can also be gripped by fear of dying. The popular notion is that dying of cancer is horribly painful. In fact, in this day and age, only a minority of cancer deaths are painful. Today's medical community is dedicated to the use of pain-killing drugs in terminal cases. However, your friend may not yet know this fact.

Fear of dying also involves fear of leaving things unfinished. If a person dies suddenly, no one expects her to have all her life and business under control. But the cancer patient, with advance warning, usually feels she must get her house in order by doing things like paying her taxes, updating her will, patching up relationships—and even cleaning her closets.

Fear of dying is *fear of mortality*. No matter how strong her faith may be, your friend isn't sure if there really is life after death. It's one thing to say so on Sunday morning—about someone else. It's another when it's about her. She can easily ask herself, "What do I need to do to get in for sure?" Answers will come—but now, only the question looms large.

So please, reach out to your friend right away. She needs the warmth of your voice, the cheer of your card, the sight of your face. Go ahead! Don't be afraid to do these "conventional" things: give a call, send a card and/or flowers, drop in for a visit. But do them with a new understanding.

Give a Call

"But I don't know what to say!" That's probably your biggest barrier as you think of calling your friend in the hospital.

Should you use the Awful Word? If not, what word should you use? "Sorry to hear of your (ulp, ah, grope, fumble) illness!" Well, maybe. Some patients might prefer that. But frankly, if you're calling me, the odds are good you know that I have cancer. So why not just say it and establish openness between us immediately? Pussyfooting around puts up a barrier between you and your friend at a time when she most needs open, honest communication.

You may also be hesitant to use the word "cancer" because you're afraid your friend might be *in denial* and you don't want to blast her out of that. Don't worry. You couldn't. If she were *in denial,* your using the word "cancer" would not be strong enough to catapult her from that stage. She will refuse to believe that she has cancer for as long as she needs to—emotionally and mentally. Only when she's ready will she move out of the *in denial* stage

"I didn't want to call and interrupt you," one friend told me. You don't have to worry. Your friend can have her calls screened if she really wants to—by nursing stations in hospitals or answering machines at home. As for being "interrupted"—that would be a delight! Think of what she's doing otherwise. She's probably lying there feeling sad, gloomy, and lonely. Your "interruption" takes her back into the real world of your everyday gossip. So pick up that phone and dial.

Send a Card

"What good is my one little card in the face of such a huge crisis?" you might be tempted to think. During my first stint in the hospital, over fifty friends, family members, colleagues, business associates, neighbors, community contacts, and friends of friends each sent me a card. Over fifty cards! What if none of them had been sent? What if each of those fifty people had thought, "Oh, what good . . . ?" I would have had zero cards instead of an abundance of them, that's what.

And don't worry about what kind to pick. Be it humorous or reflective, faith-filled or fun-filled, your choice of card reflects your special personality and reminds your friend of you. One friend sent me a cute placard of a furry critter trying with all his might to push up barbells. It read, "Give me strength!" Another friend sent me a card that read, "Have a colorful, uplifting, trust-in-Him day!"

All the cards I received filled a tote bag, and I won't get rid of them. When I was in a down mood and wondered, "Am I worth loving?"—especially during post-treatment blues—I pulled out my tote bag and knew that many people did love me.

Don't fret about how to sign off, either. Whether you sign it "yours truly," "fondly," "warmly," "as ever," "sincerely," or "love," it doesn't matter. What matters is that it comes. I used to await eagerly the daily ten o'clock mail drop. It was so encouraging to get a card.

So stop agonizing and just send your card! Your friend will be delighted. And you'll save yourself the wasted energy of feeling guilty for procrastinating.

Send Flowers

Actually, the first flowers I got were ones I sent to myself! I love flowers, and when I found out I had to go into the hospital that day, I took the time to phone for an immediate delivery. When I arrived in my room, there they were—all my favorites. I chose freesia for their fresh, sweet scent, iris for their rich color, and alstromeria—a delicate, orchid-like flower, my absolute favorite. Topped off with purple streamers, this arrangement brought exclamations from all the nurses. "Where did you get your flowers?" they asked.

I smiled and said, "I sent them to myself."

One friend, Louise, had the sensitivity to catch my "scent." She sent me just the kind of bouquet I like, full of freesia wafting their lovely perfume all over.

Michele, another friend, sent a planter. Long after its cut flowers had withered and been pulled out, the rooted green plants were still alive and growing. A powerful message of hope.

My best friend Polly sent me a bud vase—and a single fresh white or yellow rose to fill it every week I was in the hospital and at home for four months. Her message was clear. "Yes, I know it's going to be a long haul. I will help renew you each time. "

You too can be creative and intuitive in your use of flowers. And you don't have to spend a fortune. Just take some thought for your friend's preferences. Be sensitive to her sense of smell. Think about what you've seen on her table in centerpieces. Of what flower does she remind you? What message do you want to communicate through your living gift? Your gift of flowers will literally be a breath of fresh air to her.

Pay a Visit

Mary is a former college roommate who is a Ph.D. candidate at the University of Chicago. She is married and the mother of a baby boy, Joseph. But she put everything in her busy life on hold and came over to my hospital room within two hours of finding out about my cancer.

When she walked in the door, I was amazed. "Mary—what are you doing here?" I asked.

"Well, Amy, what are you doing here?" was her reply. "When I heard, I had to come," she said.

By visiting, you can help your hospitalized friend experience the virtues of life: peace, joy, hope, and love. It's hard to think these would creep into the cancer room, but they do—through you. When Polly visited me, I got peace through her eye contact. I got joy through her touch, hope through her smile. And Christ's love walked right into the room through his angel, my friend Polly.

All this happened without her saying a word. You don't necessarily have to say anything!

Ask What You Can Do

Though she really wants your help, the cancer patient herself might be shy to request it. I personally was reluctant to call some of my very closest friends—because five of them had experienced cancer losses in the recent past. I didn't want to inflict fresh pain on them. It was classic miscommunication, because they ended up hurt that I hadn't asked for their help!

Whatever the case with your friend, you may need to take the initiative and thus make it easier for her.

Asking permits your friend her freedom of choice. It gives her some sense of control in her out-of-control life.

You can use these kinds of questions to help your friend open up: "How may I help you?" This is open ended—not yes/no. If you ask, "Can I help you?" she may say, "No, that's OK." It's too easy for her to shrug you off. Open-ended questions truly invite your friend to respond to you. "What can I do for you now?" is time-limited. Because it is so immediate, it's easier for your friend to respond, "Oh—today you can buy me some cough drops. My throat's really dry."

If there's still silence in answer to your queries, make some specific, concrete offer. "I'm going to the grocery store. Is there anything I can get you?"

Again I want to urge you: don't be shy. Friendship means taking risks. It's better to take a risk than to do nothing.

Go to your friend. Reach out. Do it now.

3
Getting Prepped on Cancer Facts, Figures, and Feelings

Oncology. Metastasis. Sarcoma. Carcinoma. Adjuvant chemotherapy.

The terms flying around the cancer ward can set your head spinning. If they all sound like Greek to you, that's because about half of them are. The other half are Latin derivatives. They all add up to one big foreign language—a language you need to speak a little in order to understand and help your friend.

Reading this chapter will give you a working familiarity with cancer jargon. You'll know how to speak the basics. And you'll save your friend the trouble of educating you. You'll show her you care enough to educate yourself.

When you better understand the type of cancer your friend has, you can set more realistic expectations about the course and outcome of her disease. You'll also begin to understand where your friend might be emotionally as well as medically. Just because your Aunt Mildred had cancer doesn't mean you understand your friend's case.

Following is a glossary of cancer terms—in the order in which your friend is likely to encounter them as she goes through her cancer crisis.

Cancerspeak

Many patients who are diagnosed as having cancer go to see a doctor because of one or more of the following warning signals. Others discover they have cancer upon routine doctor visits through mammograms (breast x-rays) or stool examinations for blood. Some patients may just experience weight loss, fatigue, weakness, or a new pain.

Symptoms. The first alert your friend has is her symptoms. These will vary, of course, but the *American Cancer Society* urges people to be wary of seven warning signals:

1. Change in bowel or bladder habits
2. A sore that does not heal
3. Unusual bleeding or discharge
4. Thickening or lump in breast or elsewhere
5. Indigestion or difficulty in swallowing

6. Obvious change in wart or mole
7. Nagging cough or hoarseness

Going to the Doctor. Your friend's symptoms will motivate her to go to the doctor. She may first seek the help of her general practitioner, who will likely refer her to an oncologist— someone who specializes in cancer treatment. Oncology is from the Greek root "onkos," which means "tumor" or "mass." Or she may see a hematologist, someone who specializes in the study of blood.

Tests. The oncologist/hematologist will likely order special tests to look for suspicious growths or tissues. These tests fall into the following categories: X-ray, tests with optical instruments (endoscopy, bronchoscopy), examination of sloughed off cells (cytology), radioactive scans (nuclear medicine tests), ultrasound, CT scans (also called CAT or ACTA scans), MRI (magnetic resonance imaging), monoclonal antibodies, and biopsies.

Biopsy. The conclusive test to determine if cancer is present is the biopsy. A sample of cells is taken from the suspicious tissue, then examined and identified under a microscope.

Diagnosis. As a result of the biopsy, a diagnosis of "cancer" or "not cancer" is given.

Cancer. Your friend has received the definite diagnosis of cancer. According to the *American Cancer Society,* cancer is a large group of diseases characterized by the uncontrolled growth and spread of abnormal cells.

Cancer is malignant by definition and has the tendency to spread. A benign tumor is one which is noncancerous. It does not spread to other body parts, though it may grow. Hippocrates (about 400 B.C.) first chose the word "cancer," which means "crab" to describe malignant tumors—perhaps because the crab grabs hold and hangs onto its prey with such stubbornness.

Cancer is not just one disease. In fact, *cancer* is a generic term for a large group of diseases. Cancers behave differently depending on: 1. site of origin; 2. histologic (microscopic) types; 3. metastasis and stage of disease; 4. patient's individual genetic makeup, immune system; 5. other yet undefined factors.

Site. The chart on page 21 from *American Cancer Society* shows the incidence of cancer by site, as well as by sex. Note that the most common cancer site for women is the breast; for men, the lungs.

It is very important for you to know the site of your friend's cancer. Different sites vary vastly as to the course of the disease, treatment, and outlook for cure. Your response to your friend should be tailored to her site of cancer. "There, there, it'll be all right" might be a hopeful word to someone with skin cancer, which has an eighty-percent survival rate. But it would be cruel to pacify the person with cancer of the esophagus—a disease that has only a seven-percent rate of survival.

The chart on page 22 from the *American Cancer Society* shows the various sites of cancer and their relative five-year survival rates for the years 1977-1982.

Keep in mind that your friend's prognosis and survival with a given *one* of these cancer sites will also depend on the cell type and the stage to which the cancer has progressed. For example, while the overall figures show a thirteen-percent

Cancer Incidence by Site and Sex*
1986 Estimates

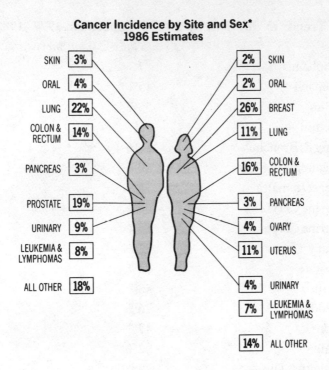

SKIN	3%		2%	SKIN
ORAL	4%		2%	ORAL
LUNG	22%		26%	BREAST
COLON & RECTUM	14%		11%	LUNG
PANCREAS	3%		16%	COLON & RECTUM
PROSTATE	19%		3%	PANCREAS
URINARY	9%		4%	OVARY
LEUKEMIA & LYMPHOMAS	8%		11%	UTERUS
ALL OTHER	18%		4%	URINARY
			7%	LEUKEMIA & LYMPHOMAS
			14%	ALL OTHER

*Excluding non-melanoma skin cancer and carcinoma in situ.

survival for lung cancer, if your friend is in an early stage of cancer such as stage 1, the survival rate may be eighty percent; but if at stage 4, zero percent. Similarly, one type of abnormal cell growth may behave very differently from another, even if they are both classified as lung cancer at the same stage!

Types of Cancer. Kinds of cancer are classified in five basic ways in the book *Choices* by Marion Morra and Eve Potts.

Trends in Survival by Site of Cancer for 1977–1982

Site	Relative 5-Year Survival %
Esophagus	7%
Stomach	15%
Colon	53%
Rectum	51%
Lung & Bronchus	13%
Melanoma of Skin	80%
Breast (female)	75%
Uterine Cervix	68%
Uterine Corpus	85%
Ovary	37%
Prostate	72%
Testis	88%
Bladder	76%
Kidney	47%
Brain	22%
Hodgkin's Disease	73%
NonHodgkin's Lymphoma	49%
Leukemia	34%

Reprinted by permission from "1986 Cancer Facts and Figures," © The American Cancer Society, Inc., *1986.*

—*Carcinomas.* These tumors begin in tissues that cover a surface or line a cavity of the body (epithelial tissues). Carcinoma is the most common type of cancer and includes lung cancer, breast cancer, colon cancer, and others.

—*Sarcomas.* These are tumors arising in the connective tissue and muscles. They attack the bone, muscle, cartilage, and lymph system. Types of sarcoma include fibrosarcoma, liposarcoma, myosarcoma, chondrosarcoma, and osteosarcoma.

—*Myelomas*. These tumors arise in the bone marrow in the blood cells that manufacture antibodies.

—*Lymphomas*. Lymphomas are cancers that originate in the lymph system—the circulatory network of vessels, spaces, and nodes carrying lymph, the almost colorless fluid that bathes the body's cells. Hodgkin's disease is one example of a lymphoma.

—*Leukemia*. This is a cancer of the blood-forming tissues (bone marrow, lymph nodes, and spleen). It is characterized by the overproduction of white blood cells.

Metastasis. The tendency of cancer to spread to other parts of the body. This is one of the most frightening aspects of cancer. Cells can break off from the original tumor, spread to other parts of the body via the bloodstream or lymphatic systems, and set up shop as yet another tumor.

No matter where it spreads, however, the cancer's designation will still be that of the original site. For example, if the cancer is initially diagnosed as cervical cancer and later spreads to the lung, it will be labeled "cervical cancer metastastized to the lung"—not "lung cancer."

Staging. At the time of diagnosis, your friend's cancer also will be described in terms of a stage. That is, to what extent has the disease metastasized? Usually the stages are 1 through 4, A or B, with 1 being the earliest, least threatening stage. Again, the cancer patient will now always be referred to by this initial stage of detection, even if the disease continues to spread.

Prognosis. Once the site of origin, the cell type, and the stage and metastasis of your friend's cancer is determined, a prognosis can be given. As we discussed previously, many factors determine your friend's prognosis and survival. The prognosis the doctor gives your friend is an estimate of what the outcome of the disease will be. It is statistical and describes what will *probably* happen to this person given what has already happened to others in the same situation.

Types of Treatment. Site, prognosis, cell type, as well as your friend's underlying physical condition and strength will determine the choices of treatment your friend will have. There are three conventional types of treatment available: surgery, radiation, and chemotherapy. (Newer, more experimental types of cancer treatment include immunotherapy, hyperthermia, and experimental combinations.)

—*Surgery.* If you hear that your friend's cancer is "inoperable," don't despair. Surgery is only one mode of treatment and can be used only on tumors in organs that can be removed without causing death. The intent of surgery is to cut out the affected area plus a safety zone around it. The colon can be removed without causing death; the liver cannot. Cancers that are "inoperable" may well be treatable by the other two means.

—*Radiation* causes tumors to shrink by destroying the cancer cells' ability to divide. Radiation can only be used on an organ that can tolerate it. Also the organ must be immovable. Radiation is generally administered in two ways— either with an external beam delivered by a machine or by radioactive material placed directly into or on the area to be treated.

24

—*Chemotherapy* kills cancer cells chemically in a number of different ways depending on what chemical is used. Chemotherapy is increasingly used in treating cancer because the drugs travel through the bloodstream. They are thus able to pursue and "catch" cancer cells wherever they have travelled within the body.

Frequently, different chemotheraphy drugs are combined in order to kill cancer cells. This process is called a "regimen" or "program." It is given in cycles in order to allow normal body tissues to recover from the effects of the drugs. Cancer cells don't recover as easily.

Chemotherapy can be given many ways: by mouth; in pill, capsule, or liquid form; intravenously as a shot or as a fluid drip; into muscles, arteries, or spinal fluid; beneath the skin; or into a body cavity such as the abdomen.

For holistic purposes, patients often add to the above treatments one or more of the following: relaxation exercises (stress management), biofeedback, macrobiotics or other special diets or vitamins, acupuncture and imagery (creative visualization), or meditation.

Multimodal Therapy. Many patients' treatment is "multimodal." This means that any or all of the above three major forms of therapy may be used. For example, if the cancer is found to be inoperable during surgery, either radiation and/or chemotherapy may be used. If all the cancer is removed by surgery, then with some types of cancer (such as breast cancer) "adjuvant" therapy (either chemotherapy or radiation or both) may be used to kill any remaining cancer cells. These cancer cells may have already spread to other parts of the body before the cancer was removed but aren't detected by the staging tests because they haven't grown significantly yet.

Outpatient versus Inpatient. Although I had all my treatment as an inpatient, chemotherapy and radiation may, depending on the patient's program, be safely administered in an outpatient clinic or office. Your friend's physician will know if this is feasible. If your friend receives treatment as an outpatient, premedication to prevent nausea may make her very sleepy. Make sure she has a ride to and from the doctor.

Side Effects. The *National Cancer Institute* publishes two excellent booklets on different cancer treatments as well as the side effects—"Chemotherapy and You," and "Radiation Therapy and You." Side effects are common but not unmanageable. They may range from nothing more than a little nausea to more intense nausea and vomiting. Your friend may be generally tired and more prone to infections than usual.

Cancer Treatment Protocols. I was involved in an experimental protocol. Because the number of people with cancer is growing every year and the cause is still largely unknown, the *National Cancer Institute* approves of and gives funding to the multitude of cancer treatment studies going on around the country. Your friend should be encouraged to ask her oncologist to explain all her treatment options available for her stage and type of cancer. If there is already a moderately effective treatment for her cancer, then a program will be set up to improve on it; if none is available (your friend may technically have a zero-percent cure rate according to the chart), then the doctors will set up a new experimental approach for the patient.

Recurrence. Recurrence is the reappearance of the same type of cancer at the same place, nearby (regional), or at a distant body location (metastasis). Remission or cure? When can one say cancer is cured? That is the question that will continue to haunt your friend once her treatment is complete. The answer depends upon the original site and stage of the cancer, as well as other factors. It may be anywhere from two to fifteen years. Until that time, if no further symptoms show up, the most that can be said is that the patient is in remission. In other words, *limbo*.

To get information about the type of cancer your friend has and about its likely treatment, you can call these toll-free numbers and request the free literature offered by:

The *American Cancer Society* (a private nonprofit organization)
1 (800) ACS–2345

The *Cancer Information Service* (coordinated by the National Cancer Institute, part of the U.S. Department of Health and Human Services)
1 (800) 4–CANCER

Amy's Story
My personal cancer story took this shape. I experienced vaginal bleeding for six weeks, which prompted me to see a gynecologist. His recommendation was to go off the hormonal treatment I was on at the time. His opinion was that the bleeding was due to stress—I had recently undergone knee surgery and came to his office in a leg cast and using crutches.

After I continued to bleed for another two months, I returned, and he performed a "Pap" test. It was negative, like all my previous routine, twice-a-year "Pap" tests. But I continued to bleed for two more months, at which point the doctor did a uterine biopsy, which was also negative. He then decided I should take a hormone prescription to correct the bleeding.

By this point, however, I had lost trust in this physician and sought a second opinion. The second physician promptly sent me to an oncologist, who did a colposcopy, a test by which the cervix can be examined for any suspicious-looking cells. A biopsy was also performed. Because I was by this time bleeding profusely, with large, heavy clots, the oncologist admitted me to the hospital as an emergency patient.

The next day he gave me my diagnosis: cancer of the cervix.

To assess the metastasis, if any, and determine the staging, I was given further tests including a CAT scan, and (to check for cancer in the rectum) a barium enema X-ray. I also underwent exploratory surgery to look for any spread of cancer and to conduct a cystoscopy (to check for cancer in the bladder).

When my cancer was first detected, I was staged as a 1-B, a tumor that had not spread to other organs. With the staging of 1-B, I was given a cure prognosis of eighty percent. The treatment recommended was surgery—removal of my uterus, ovaries, and Fallopian tubes.

But the surgery included the examination of lymph nodes in the pelvic area. Unfortunately, cancer was found in some of these nodes, so the physicians decided to change the treatment plan and removed only the ovaries and Fallopian tubes, leaving the uterus available for radiation treatment.

When I woke up, my physician notified me of the findings— that the cancer had spread to some lymph nodes on one side of the pelvic area. As a result, he told me, my cure prognosis had now dropped to fifty percent. He encouraged a radiation treatment plan.

However, a few days later, while I was still in the hospital recovering from my surgery, further biopsies of other nodes that were removed disclosed that the lymph nodes on both sides of the pelvic cavity were involved. My physician told me that my cure prognosis had now dropped to less than thirty percent. It was then I asked a blunt question, and received an equally blunt reply. "Who in your personal experience has lived to the five-year mark with my type and spread of cancer?" I asked my doctor.

"No one," he replied.

I signed up for an experimental treatment protocol as a result of that news. I had had a minor operation to implant a portacatheter under the skin on my chest to receive the IV. It helped avoid being pricked every day.

My treatment plan repeated the following cycle five times. On Sunday night I'd check into the hospital and receive, through an IV, a chemotherapy drug called cisplatinum. Monday through Friday I received radiation treatments twice a day—one in the morning, one in the afternoon. I received a twenty-four-hour-a-day intravenous drip of another chemotherapy drug, 5-FU. Saturday morning I would go home for a week of what was euphemistically called "R and R," to return the following Sunday evening and start over again.

My five week-on/week-off treatments concluded with another type of radiation treatment: a radiation implant. Under anesthesia, radioactive pellets were inserted into my cervix. Of necessity I was then put in isolation for three days.

Such an aggressive course of treatment exacts a toll.

The initial cisplatinum caused such nausea that whatever I had to eat Sunday morning I would lose Sunday evening. I remember having Sunday brunch at the Ritz and asking myself *why*—but it did taste wonderful, whatever its future!

Chemotherapy also produced great fatigue.

The short-term result of radiation was the constriction of the vaginal wall, resulting in the loss of some sensation. Studies show that women who have received radiation treatments have more negative sexual attitudes and performance than those who have had only surgery, and that their partners also respond more negatively, mistakenly fearing radiation contamination.

During the week "between" treatments, I continued to be both tired and nauseated—and very attached to the bathroom because of irritable-bowel syndrome, also a result of radiation.

Yet somehow in the midst of all my treatment, I managed to find a streak of wry humor. I imagined playing connect-the-dots with my scar tissue and my iodine dots for placement of radiation. I remembered Robert Schuller saying, "Turn your scars into stars." My paraphrase became, "Turn your scars into connect-the-dots." I thought a lot about this when I was alone for three days, immobilized in bed with the radiation implant.

I am still experiencing, though, the serious continuing results of my treatment. The long-term effects of radiation are un-known. But within six months of my treatment I developed proctitis, which includes minor rectal bleeding, probably a consequence of the aggressive radiation I received. Fifteen months later I developed cystitis, a bladder condition that is also probably a result of the radiation.

I've certainly been frightened with each new quirk, wonder-ing if it were the reappearance of cancer. Luckily both the rectal and urinary bleeding are "just" long-term radiation dam-age. Today, when people ask me, "Are you in remission?" I have to say, "Yes. I'm symptom-free." But I am in limbo as well.

The Emotional Rollercoaster

Once your friend has been diagnosed with cancer, she steps onto an emotional rollercoaster ride that is not fun. Dr. James R. Hodge, chairman of the Department of Psychiatry at the Akron City Hospital, Akron, Ohio, describes what this roller-coaster ride can be like from firsthand experience: his own wife was diagnosed with cancer several years ago. This emotional sequence was first described by Dr. Elisabeth Kübler-Ross in her monumental work on death and dying.

Shock, surprise, and fear are the first plunge on this no-fun ride. Even though your friend may have been expecting it, the news still leaves her numb. You may tell her something one day and find you need to repeat exactly the same information the next.

Then, says Hodge, the patient attempts to find emotional release by trying to pretend this really isn't happening to her. But reality won't go away, and soon she finds she must decide whom to tell. She must also decide who she can trust with her feelings of anger, depression, anxiety, and despair. If you are able to hear these feelings you will be of great help to her.

As anxiety sets in, the patient will imagine exaggerated physical symptoms: the lump seems bigger, the bleeding seems worse.

The anxiety can turn into panic. The patient may become obsessed with thinking about her cancer and may be convinced it has already spread throughout her entire body. "The patient is suffering severely," says Hodge. "Often, merely prescribing that he ventilate his panic is enough, but there has to be someone . . . to whom he can ventilate." That person can be you—the friend.

As the patient wears herself out with panic, guilt sets in.

She may begin to wonder what she did to deserve this.

"Sometimes these guilt feelings become strong enough to cause suicide," states Hodge. Your gentle reassurance that cancer is not punishment, and that God truly loves her can help your friend roll with this phase of the ride.

After feeling guilty and blaming herself, the patient gets angry and blames others—often including God. This anger is healthy, because it's a form of energy. But don't be surprised if some of it gets irrationally directed at you.

Next, the patient may try bargaining, especially with God. "If you keep me alive, I'll give my life completely to you." When she sees the futility of bargaining, the patient may become depressed, thinking that she might just as well give up and die. This is a very dangerous stage that may occur after major surgery and during radiation or chemotherapy. Your friend needs encouragement, and may even need professional psychotherapy in dealing with her depression. "Without it, [she] may not take the treatment which may preserve life," says Hodge.

Then there can be a stage of adjustment to the reality of living with cancer, and to active participation in the treatment. The patient says to herself, "I've looked at the alternatives and I see my choices clearly. I will take the treatment. I will live till I die. And I will make the most of it."

Finally, concludes Hodges, after the five years (or whatever time frame the doctor has set), your friend can think of herself as a former cancer patient—a survivor—even though she knows there are still no guarantees.

If it sounds like a tall order for a friend to hang on through this emotional rollercoaster, I guess it is. But be assured: you can only do what you can do. In her heart, your friend knows this. And though it's hard to read about some of these predictable ups and downs, the knowledge will make them less surprising to you when your friend exhibits them. And when you do! You'll be having your own emotional ups and downs—not necessarily at the same time or in the same sequence as your friend. In fact, don't be surprised if it takes you longer to get to reach the stage of acceptance than it does your friend!

A final reminder about the emotional rollercoaster, one that I can't repeat too often. Be sure to take time out for yourself. No, your friend can't get off the rollercoaster ride. But you can. You owe it to yourself—and to her—to get off often enough to keep yourself refreshed.

Applying Your Findings to Your Friend

Cancer strikes individuals. While most people will go through some form of the above emotional rollercoaster, other factors will enter into the particular ways the disease impacts your friend.

When I was diagnosed with cancer, I was the "typical" young career woman. Single, without children, I was in my seventh year as an independent management consultant, specializing in training executives and business professionals in how to make successful proposals and presentations. Cancer has affected me directly in all areas of my life. I can neither conceive nor adopt children. And with such a prognosis, who would want to love me, bond, or mate? And I, too, share concern about the job discrimination experienced by most cancer patients.

As you think of your friend, consider what life issues her

cancer will affect. Appropriately, doctors think of cells and causes when they say "cancer." But patients often consider consequences and costs—financial and emotional—when they think of cancer.

Cancer also touches an individual's faith. How has your friend responded to previous life crises? Has her faith been strengthened? Or has it tended to fall apart?

For me, looking at my own history of dealing with crises gave me confidence. I saw that my faith had stood the test of previous loss.

I have a card that was given to me during a prior crisis. I framed it and hung it by my key rack where I could see it every day. It still provides me with strength and insight. Written by author Louise Haskins, it reads, "And I said to the man who stood at the gate of the year, 'Give me a light that I may tread safely into the unknown.' And he replied, 'Go out into the darkness and put thine hand into the hand of God. That shall be to thee better than light and safer than a known way.' "

As a cancer patient, I wanted to know everything. Every nuance of my condition. Every possible impact of every possible treatment. But that was not the answer, as it had not been the answer in past crises. The answer is to put my hand into God's hand. That is safer . . . and much better.

4
Offering Your Helping Hands

You've done some homework now and are starting to understand the nature of your friend's illness. You feel ready to do some down-to-earth practical helping. But what can you do? There's so much she needs—and you have only two hands!

Yes, two hands. Like the card you sent, which became part of the flood of over fifty cards, your two hands are not the only ones God will use to care for your friend. God has many hands. Each pair will do something different—something only they can do. But together, all the hands will make up God's cosmic care plan for your friend.

So let your hands do their special task. Trust your impulses. What do you feel like doing for your friend? What comes naturally to you? Trust that God is the originator of that nudge.

Following are only a few of the many things my friends did for me during my five-month treatment. I describe them to express my deep thankfulness to these friends. I also wish to demonstrate to you the range of gifts possible—and how together they can form a wealth of caring. I don't want to impose any "shoulds" on you. Instead, I hope you will use these as thought-joggers for your own special contribution. Borrow a little of this and a little of that—or spin off in a completely new direction.

Whatever you do, I hope you will be inspired to extend your helping hands. The value of any gift is impossible to measure. So don't screen out what you think you can and can't do. Offer your gift.

Case Studies in Caring

Certain friends offered me so many gifts that are interwoven with my life that I have chosen to describe them in "case studies." Though the caring my friends offered was tailored to my status as a single career woman, you will discover many ways of caring that any cancer patient needs.

Twenty-four-hour availability. Polly and Tom were gracious enough to offer me 24-hour access to their lives, both in their home and at their business. What a gift for a single, self-employed person such as myself!

Their sofa was my favorite place to stay, and they let me— even though this meant disrupting their whole household routine! But the view from that sofa is so wonderful. Polly and Tom's house is situated right on the Fox River. From the sofa, when I woke up, I could see the morning sun glittering on the slow-flowing water. Bicyclists glided by on the riverside bike path. Ducks waddled on the lawn. It was both homey and heavenly.

Polly and Tom also made me welcome to hang out in their showroom at the Merchandise Mart, where a steady stream of people flows in and out all day long. This was a wonderful social outlet for me. There I could temporarily shed my cancer identity and chit-chat with the customers.

Polly and Tom also offered me a get-away refuge—their guest house on Captiva Island. This is the same island on which Anne Morrow Lindbergh wrote her famous *Gift from the Sea*. Polly and Tom's house is only a block from the Gulf on this vegetated and tropical paradise where key lime and orange trees bloom, hibiscus wraps itself around the house, the scheffleras soar high and green, and the stars really do twinkle at night. Here was a haven for solitude, reflection, and prayer— an atmosphere that breathed nature's healing.

Tom's special gift to me was time with Polly. He encouraged her to attend to me. I felt his care in this sacrifice of sharing. Because of his generosity, Polly could do things like spending the night with me when I needed company.

"Nest and tuck" time. I had a "nesting place" with my friends Rae and Bill, whose home was also a haven to me. Their house has sixty-foot-wide sliding glass doors that open onto a beautiful meadow. From the deck that overlooks the meadow I could hear all the sounds of the birds. Squirrels would clamber up. Rabbits would hop in the brambles.

At night, Rae would tuck me in and kiss me on the cheeks and eyelids. On the nightstand were mystery books, my favorite, and graham crackers with milk or hot chocolate. This was real nest and tuck time. It felt OK to be treated just as I was—a vulnerable, hurting child.

Rae "nested" me in the hospital, too. She gave me a stuffed toy cat that was a perfect look-alike for one of my cats. When I took that stuffed cat to the hospital I was bringing with me a piece of my home—my critters.

Caring across the miles. My friend Pat is an eloquent witness to how much caring can be done long distance. Though once a fellow church member, Pat had moved to New Jersey by the time my cancer struck.

"Amy," Pat told me in a phone conversation after my five-month treatment ordeal was over, "you made it easy for your friends to take care of you."

"I did?" I said.

"Yes," said Pat with a big grin. "You assigned us duties. You told me, 'You are the card lady!' "

Maybe so. But Pat did her duty to a "T." She sent cards faithfully every couple of days. They were always signed, "Love you, Pat." She also solicited her mother Kay and her daughter Sheri to join the effort.

But that's not all. In cahoots with Polly, Pat rented a clown to come to the hospital with bright, colorful helium balloons. Half of them had "Amy" on them! The other half said, "I love you." Those joyous balloons were a wonderful, blatant denial of the automatic doom and gloom associated with the diagnosis of cancer. They added a welcome contrast to the sterility of the hospital decor. I tied the balloons to the night stand where they could blow in the vent, a bright streamer of color.

Pat also sent to the hospital what I call my "beauty basket." It was a beautiful basket full of goodies.

There were lotions—apricot, aloe, and others to soothe my parched skin.

There was a rose-colored tea cup and saucer with herb teas

and cinnamon sticks. What a delight for me! I couldn't eat much but I really enjoyed some teas.

There was a four-inch tall statue of three seagulls flying. A sort of "Jonathan Livingston Seagull" piece.

And there was what I came to think of as my "footprint memento." It was a cleaned-up spice jar filled with sand and shells and tied with a delicate pink ribbon. Pat sent it to remind me of the time she and I spent doing cartwheels down the shore. But I also took it as a reminder of the poem "Footprints," in which the poet imagines Jesus picking him up and carrying him through a crisis. Gifts given with one intention can have multiple meanings and associations.

A Checklist of Caring

As your friend goes through her treatment, she needs you to lift her spirits. There are so many things you can do that have this "uplift" effect. As you mull over what your special gift might be, take some cues from this checklist. And remember: so often, the very thing you think "Oh, I shouldn't" or "Oh, no—not that!" may be exactly what your cancer patient friend needs. She wants you to celebrate life with her!

While she's in the hospital:
—*Bring children.* When my high school friend Carolyn came to visit me in the hospital, her two beautiful children accompanied her—Abigail, age three, and Lydia, nine months. Together we went to the tea room, where Abigail presented me with a handmade card.

No doubt Carolyn had wondered about bringing her babies. "Is it fair to parade my two beautiful children in front of you, Amy?" If she would have asked me, my answer certainly would have been, "You bet!" I'm so glad she followed her intuition! Those children brought life to me.

—*Share photos of past memories.* Peggy was part of the group I toured the Holy Land with. When she heard of my illness, she made a set of pictures of our tour and sent them to me. Those photos brought back such great memories of being loved and of having fellowship with the Lord.

Some people might fear it would be morbid to stir up memories of past happiness. But those photos and the memories they contained were nothing but uplifting for me. They sounded a note of hope, as I thought, "See— God took care of you on that trip to the Middle East! He'll take care of you now."

—*Check-in with phone calls.* Polly gave me good morning and good night phone calls every day I was in the hospital. Was that ever wonderful!

—*Give encouraging tapes.* Find out if your friend has a tape recorder. If not, go together with several others and buy an inexpensive one, now available for as low as $29.

Then lend your friend tapes. Borrow Christian teaching tapes from your church's library, get or make tapes of the pastor's sermons, and check the public library for condensed or unabridged readings of books.

—*Give music.* Once you've given your friend the tape recorder, don't forget how soothing and uplifting music can be!

My mother sent me a tape of Dame Kiri Te Kanawa singing many beautiful and spiritually exalting pieces.

Another friend, Janet, gave me Amy Grant's *Age to Age,* which turned out to be a great favorite.

—*Keep your friend in touch with the everyday.* It's so important for your friend to feel like part of the everyday world. Several people helped me stay in tune—my father by sending newspaper clippings or church bulletin snippets, Polly by sending cartoons.

—*Make something happen—now.* Another friend named Tom brought me an instant lottery ticket—and that generated so much fun for me! It was "Get ready, get set, go!"— scrape off the silver, and something can happen right now! In fact, it did—I won two dollars. Big deal, right? But it was, because it really broke the routine.

—*Take dictation.* I had tons of thank-you notes that needed to be written, and I was given lovely note cards and postage. But I couldn't focus well enough to do them myself. I didn't think of it at the time, but a friend could have taken dictation and written them for me.

—*Read to your friend.* Read to me, please—especially my *Forward Day by Day,* my daily Bible readings guide. I was snipped, zapped, and so exhausted I couldn't even look at TV, let alone the printed words on a page.

—*Keep your friend in touch with nature.* Sylvia sent me a card in which she had pressed several dried fall leaves she collected on a walk. Those leaves were wonderful— they made me want to go and kick through them again when I could.

—*Do errands or chores.* Work-related or personal, there's a host of things you can do. Try these:

> water my plants
> watch over and take care of my house or apartment
> go to the dry cleaner or the shoe repair

get my car washed and/or the gas tank filled
bring mail to the hospital
Federal express something for my job
get something Xeroxed

—*Send a mascot for memories.* The mascot of St. Mark's
Episcopal church is a lion. Donna, the rector's wife and
a member of the church's St. Margaret's Guild, sent me
a little stuffed lion to be my personal mascot and remind
me of all those caring, loving people in that church.

—*Give your friend something to hug.* Karen, an acquaintance,
sent a teddy bear to the hospital. Not only was it very
huggable, but it helped me realize that I'd been a significant person in her faith journey.

—*Give your friend Scripture.* Virginia gave me the gift of
Scripture—and she did it in a special way. Instead of just
plopping a couple references on a card and expecting me
to haul out my Bible and fumble through it, she took the
time to write the passages out in full. Here are the texts
she shared with me:

"My grace is sufficient for you, for my power is made
perfect in weakness" (2 Corinthians 12:9, NIV).

"[He] is able to do immeasurably more than all we ask
or imagine, according to his power that is at work within
us" (Ephesians 3:20, NIV).

"God is our refuge and strength, an ever present help
in trouble. Therefore we will not fear, though the earth
give way and the mountains fall into the heart of the sea,
though its waters roar and foam and the mountains quake
with their surging" (Psalm 46:1-3, NIV).

42

—*Send books.* There are so many different kinds of books you can send your friend! There are inspirational books, teaching books, and humorous ones. Though she may not be able to read them right now, the books will give your friend something to look forward to.

One of my favorite inspirational books was *Growing Into the Blue* by Ulrich Schaffer, a gift from my friend Linda. This lovely photo-poetry book gave me double delight. The first time through, I just looked at the beautiful pictures and was brought in touch with nature. The second time through, I enjoyed the poetry.

Sylvia sent me a rainbow-colored card/book called *Faith Is* by Pamela Reeve. The title of that book showed me that Sylvia realized cancer was affecting my faith as well as my life, and she wasn't shy about saying so.

Her inscription was very special to me. "Dear Amy," it read. "This little book has become very precious to me. No matter what day it is or what is facing me, I find peace just reading it."

Faith is a black leather-bound Bible, yes. But thanks to Sylvia's gift, it's also a rainbow of color.

Karolee sent me the book *You Gotta Keep Dancin'* by Tim Hansel. It brought a welcome dose of optimism.

A former mentor of mine, Frances, sent me two very significant educational books. *Anatomy of an Illness* by Norman Cousins, is a classic on positive thinking as an effective adjunct to treatment. Cousins really believes in laughter as a healing force. *Getting Well Again,* by Drs. Simonton and Simonton, is the classic book about visualizing health and healing. Through these books, Frances was saying to me, "Amy, you've got cancer. Fight it!" I really appreciated her firm pragmatism.

Don't overlook humorous books, or just plain old best-sellers or diversionary books. My particular passion happens to be mysteries, and Louise was a great one for passing those along.

And along with the book, why not tuck in a bookmarker? Joyce gave me one that says simply, "Jesus loves me"—and I love it.

When your friend is out of the hospital (or between stays):

—*Invite her out for dinner.* Most people automatically think "chemotherapy = don't eat!" Not so for me! Gourmet dining is one of my greatest pleasures in life, and my friend David knew it. So he kept our dinner dates during my off-treatment weeks. This helped me retain my sense of enjoyment in something I normally take pleasure in. At least I could savor the four-star ambience.

—*Give subscriptions.* Donna gave me a subscription to *The Anglican Digest;* Joyce gave me the *Daily Word.*

A gift subscription to *Coping* could be wonderful for your friend. *Coping* is a publication written for a lay audience. It provides inspiration and information for cancer patients and their families on the art of living with cancer, and features articles on insurance, drugs, lifestyles, prevention, and other topics. Address subscription correspondence to *Coping,* P.O. Box 54693, Boulder, CO 80322, or call 1 (800) 525-0643.

—*Be personal.* Theresa is an artist living in San Francisco. She painted a picture of my essence, which she called my "Vessel." Its fiery dynamism continues to inspire me from its place on my office wall.

—Give a donation. I was profoundly moved when I received a card saying that Evan had made a donation to the *American Cancer Society* in my name.

—Give a piece of home. Melba sent me a special care package of homemade cookies and other edibles. Such thoughtfulness was truly special.

—Invite your friend out. Joe is a delightful, lovable seventy-year-old man whose wife had died following a bout with cancer six months previously. He would take me out to dinner every so often and tell me tales of world travels and going fishing with his grandson in Canada. How wonderful it was to dress, dine, and listen to beautiful stories. I hope it was as therapeutic for him as it was for me.

—Keep previous dates (if possible). Polly and I had had a longstanding date for a bed-and-breakfast weekend in scenic Galena. We kept it, and it was a lovely fall nature weekend. We walked through parks overlooking the winding Mississippi, looked at antiques, and toured the home of General Ulysses S. Grant.

—Include your friend in outings (if she's able). Diane invited me to a fall picnic day in the country. She was inviting her father, Bill and his wife Rae, and went a step further to say, "Is Amy out of the hospital? I think she would enjoy this!" And I certainly did! The picnic was a three-family affair, complete with teenagers. It was on Jim and Dee's farm in a beautiful area of ravines and pine trees. We enjoyed a classic hot dog, hamburger, baked beans, and potato salad picnic, complete with swatting the flies and killing the mosquitoes. Then we took a tour to see the pigs the farm raised—from cute little oinkers to big

snouters. The whole day was wonderful!

Gifts from business associates and service people. If you are a business associate or a service acquaintance, your gifts count also! So please give them.

Marilyn, who owns the secretarial service I use, offered me the gift of flexibility. On two occasions when I was feeling OK, she adapted her working schedule to my ability to work, even at off-hours.

Larry, a former boss, called me up during my treatment off-week, said, "I'd love to visit," and set up a business break-fast. He was just doing what he'd naturally do—but it gave me such a sense of "business as usual"—just like in the good old days.

Nicholas is a major client. He not only rescheduled our work around my health, but he and his wife were able to talk to me about cancer and work-related subjects, like how to handle work discrimination.

Bill is also a major client. As my cancer crisis deepened throughout the first week after my emergency admit, I had to call him and postpone three separate times. Each time, he gave me great assurance to devote my energies to getting well. He also asked if he should pass on the info to his colleagues. I said yes, and as a result, received more lovely cards, calls, and flowers.

Maureen and Tracy, two other clients—both of whom had cancer in their family histories—reminded me of the impor-tance of focusing on living—not just working. It was an impor-tant word for someone like me who tends to think, "But work is my life!"

Lorie runs the kennel where I board my cats. She told me,

"For you, we'll stretch the arrival and departure times for the cats." That little extra bit of service became a gift.

I've experienced similar care from other service people. The dry cleaner told me, "Usually we don't deliver. But for you, I'll personally deliver your clothes. Don't worry!"

The Good Grapevine

There's one final thing you can do for your cancer patient friend. You can prayerfully and discreetly pass on news of her illness to other helpers.

"Should I pass this on?" is definitely a big question. But my answer, especially within the Church, is yes. But always ask permission, again letting your friend maintain a sense of control. By passing on the news to appropriate people, you multiply your friend's chances of receiving caring support and prayer. Not only that, but the good grapevine spares your friend from always having to be the one to break the news. That can be a relief.

Let me share a few examples from my own experience.

My former church asked me first, then announced in the bulletin so people could pray for me: "Former parishioner Amy Harwell is in St. Luke's with cancer." The good grapevine went into effect. A parishioner told a Christian nurse who worked at St. Luke's. That nurse took her own off-duty time and came and prayed with me!

My father also did some good grapevining. He ran into some former business associates who attended my childhood church, St. Peter's United Church of Christ. These business associates passed on the news to my former minister, Bob, and he came to visit me in the hospital.

I can't close this chapter without sharing one more delightful example of how God set into effect his very own cosmic care plan for me. As you recall, I had designated Pat to be "the card lady." But I hadn't counted on "God's letter writer." Janet was really just an acquaintance from St. Mark's when she began sending me cards—so regularly and faithfully that I felt almost guilty to receive such beneficence. Her cards were easily spottable in my mail—two-by-three-inch envelopes. They were always signed, "Praying for you, Love, Janet."

And she just kept sending them!

I finally felt I had to alert her when I was out of my crisis, so that she could pass her love along to the next person in crisis. In effect I was telling her, "You have limited resources."

How foolish of me! Who am I to tell her she had limited resources? Who am I to say, "You can't love me?" Fortunately, I finally wised up and continued to receive her love.

Janet and I had a good laugh over this a year later when I led an adult discussion group at St. Mark's. I told the group what a great thing it had been to receive all those cards from everyone. Then I said, "And there's one in our midst who has been just overwhelming!" Janet piped up and said, "And she told me to stop!"

Support and Relieve the Caregiver

As you offer your helping hands to your friend, don't overlook the person who is the major caregiver in her life. He or she needs some uplifting, too!

My parents, who qualify as my primary caregivers (since I am single), live 700 miles away. Although they would have moved for the entire time, I felt more comfortable asking them to come for several visits throughout my treatment. If I could have changed any one thing in my crisis, I would have wanted to rally more support for my parents. They needed care, too. This need for support is true of all spouses, parents, and children—or whomever is the primary caregiver. At least I got fussed over, and it was expected for me to have ups and downs. At least I could participate in my treatment—I was doing something. But their pains and aches of watching me lacked the embrace of caring others.

I was thankful for the times my friends would join them in the hospital tea room, or sit side by side in the family lounge during some of my tougher ordeals.

The primary caregiver needs to be cared for. Support them so they can dedicate their energies to caring for their own loved one. Go in and do their work for them. Mow the lawn, drive the kids to lessons, vacuum the house, load and unload the dishwasher.

Give them some play time. Go out to a movie or dinner with them. Play golf. Shop for something special. The primary caretaker has a need to take time out.

Networking to Other Resources

When your friend is in the hospital she is under 24-hour-a-day care and supervision. When I was in the hospital, a nurse named Donnette "adopted" me. Full of TLC, she demonstrated what every cancer patient knows—how important nurses are for emotional as well as physical care. If your friend is lucky, she also will have her "Donnettes." But when your friend gets out of the hospital, there is no longer anyone in charge of her physical care—or her emotional well-being.

You may want to suggest that she link up with other resources to help her through this time. Possible services to connect her with include the following:

Professional counseling. Hospital social workers, chaplains, and other specially trained psychologists or psychiatrists can provide an important lifeline. My own full-service oncology team included (in addition to my surgeon, radiologist, and chemotherapist) a psychiatrist, who offered some helpful advice for the difficult times.

General rehabilitation services. The *American Cancer Society* offers transportation service, equipment, dressings, and the like.

Educational services. The "I Can Cope" seminar, co-sponsored by the *American Cancer Society* and local hospitals, is an educational course designed to help patients and family members cope with cancer, including its impact on emotions, self-esteem, sexuality, and other life issues. You can find out more about this course by calling 1 (800) ACS–2345.

My mother took the course in her home location of Florida. Unfortunately, it wasn't available for me in Chicago at the time, or we would have benefitted greatly from discussing the material via phone. But it was a great comfort to me to know that she cared enough to get informed.

Support groups. "Make Today Count," "Y-Me" (for breast cancer patients), the "Ostomy Club," and "Spirit and Breath," are a few of the local programs that provide support. Usually they are listed with the *American Cancer Society* units in your area.

Patient visitor program. A patient visitor is a specially trained volunteer visitor who has successfully recovered from cancer treatment and who volunteers time to meet and share experiences with current cancer patients. Writing in the *Journal of MAG,* Susan Connelly (M.S.W., A.C.S.W.) says, "Patient visitors relate to the person behind the diagnosis, thereby decreasing the loneliness and alienation felt by many cancer patients."

Some patient visitors are matched by cancer site. "CanSurmount" is an *American Cancer Society* program that provides patient visitors on a non-site specific basis.

Hospice. If appropriate, you may suggest hospice care for your friend. Hospice is an alternative to aggressive therapy for terminal patients—those expected to die within six months—which accents care, not cure.

When I learned that my friend Shirley's father-in-law had been diagnosed with lung cancer, I shot off a note suggesting she look into hospice. Shirley took the suggestion and contacted one. Her father-in-law died three months later, at home, in the company of his wife and under the care of a hospice team.

Patient to patient. Network your own support system. Link up your friend—with her permission of course—with someone you know who is comfortable sharing her experience.

The real estate woman in my office building provided this kind of networking. After getting my OK, she gave my name to a woman named Patty, who had just been diagnosed with lung cancer.

As a result of the real estate woman's initiative, I was able to help Patty. I visited her in her home and in the hospital, answered some of her questions about treatment, passed on books that had helped me, looked into head coverings such as wigs, called periodically, and recommended *Cope Magazine*.

This Christmas, I got a thank-you note from Patty. It read, "Thank you for your support in my 'fight.' It means the world to me. I know that you understand that. I guess that's what makes you so special. Thank you for being there!" With the note was a gift—a crystal butterfly candy dish. Patty told me,

"I had to buy you this gift—because you're that butterfly."

Literature. Check the public library, bookstores, and your church library for books and articles you think might be helpful to your friend.

After I left the hospital the first time, I went to my church, Fourth Presbyterian, and found in the library two autobiographies and a book on the cancer patient. The autobiographies, especially, ministered to me, because at the time I did not personally know anyone who had cancer.

There are so many things your helping hands can do! You will never know what part your gift will play in your friend's life. But you can know that you are part of God's cosmic care plan for her.

5
Sharing
Your Healing
Heart

"The best and most beautiful things in the world cannot be seen or even touched," said Helen Keller. "They must be felt with the heart."

There is one more precious gift some of you will be called on to give: the gift of your healing heart.

The cancer patient's primary goal is to reach acceptance of her present condition so she can commit her energies to getting better—however she defines that. Her diagnosis has backed her up against the wall with the question, "Why me?" In her treatment, she has chosen to accept upfront damage—physical, emotional, and financial—as the price she pays for more time to live. However, she does not feel like the whole, well, normal person she once was.

Ultimately, of course, your friend must get her sense of

wholeness from God and her relationship with him. But she experiences part of God's loving acceptance through the care of his "angels on earth"—people like you. Distinguished theologian Martin Marty has remarked that the line is as much "What a Jesus we have in a friend" as "What a friend we have in Jesus." I have found that to be very true.

The question is, then, will my friends acknowledge their God-inspired inner impulse that says, "Go to her. Do not avoid her"? Don't let your fear of sickness and dying prevent you from gaining the blessing of sharing your healing heart.

This is not necessarily something that has to take loads of time. Many professional counseling sessions are only 45 minutes once a week—most are never longer than an hour.

"But," you say, "I'm not a trained counselor!"

Although you cannot replace a professional counselor, if your friend's depression deepens to the point where she needs one, there is much that you can do.

You see, it is not so much a matter of "correct technique." It's not *what you say* that counts. It is *what your friend says*. Being a good listener is what's important. You need to be content with few answers and let her seek her own answers.

What is a healing heart? When it was offered to me, I couldn't touch it. I couldn't hold it. I couldn't see it. But I felt the healing hearts of my friends as they used their helping skills to listen, question, touch, and pray.

Listening

A *talker* comes within my personal boundary needing me.

A *listener* comes to me with this gift: "You are more important to me right now than any other item on the docket—my business dealings, my Christmas shopping, a letter that must be written."

If I am worth more than these things, I must really have value!

A *talker* bombards me with her stories, her pain, her "I can top that one." She can't stand the silences.

A *listener* listens to me. She listens with her body. She listens with her heart. She can bear the silences. She can hear what actress Jill Ireland calls the patient's "toxic energy." Writing in her recent cancer autobiography, Ireland says, "It's a shame you can't just talk to the wall and get rid of [the toxic energy], but there has to be a receiver. You have to talk out your horrible, bad feelings. Somebody has to receive them . . . The right therapist or the right friend is vital."

With your body. "A listener needs to look the part," says John W. Drakeford in his book *The Awesome Power of the Listening Heart*. Since studies suggest that ninety-three percent of communication is nonverbal, Drakeford describes body postures that say, "I'm listening." From head to toe, your whole bearing can communicate openness—or closedness.

—*Head*. Tilt your head like a sunflower toward the person. Nod from time to time as appropriate.

—*Eyes*. Maintain a comfortable level of eye contact. Of course, some people cannot tolerate a direct gaze, nor can you maintain one indefinitely. In that case, try looking just over your friend's shoulder. This will demonstrate your care without staring.

—*Mouth*. Smile, or maintain a relaxed position of your lips. Pursed or tightened lips can be interpreted as disapproval.

—*Torso*. Lean forward toward your friend to indicate your interest and concern. Leaning back or away consistently could express avoidance, whether conscious or subconscious. Remember she is already worried about her acceptability.

—*Arms*. Maintain an open posture of arms uncrossed, resting comfortably at your sides. Crossing your arms over your chest could be interpreted as a defensive posture. If appropriate, you might hold your friend's hand, or rest your arm nearby—like a cat reaching out a love-pat paw.

With your heart. Listen to your friend for feelings, not just for facts. Though she may not express them in so many words, what emotions are lurking below the surface of her talk?

A technique called "active listening" invites us to reflect or feed back to our friend what we think we're hearing. "Sounds like you're frightened that you will lose your job because of this cancer." If your friend disagrees with your interpretation, let it go. It's not your job to push your hypothesis on her. And *never* negate any direct expression of feeling. "I'm afraid," your friend says. "Oh, don't be afraid" is the wrong response because it cuts off further honest communication of feeling. Instead, acknowledge feeling. "Yes, I can understand why you would feel frightened."

My friends Louise and Harvey are beautiful listeners. They offered me an opportunity to unload my deep philosophical concerns. They didn't run from that kind of heavy discussion. With them, it wasn't just a "Hi, how are you?" They listened to and discussed my burning questions: "What does my cancer mean? Is it punishment? Is it a result of my repressing anger?"

With them I worked through the "why" of my cancer—and my ability to accept myself as I was with cancer. When Harvey, a former professor at the University of Chicago, did talk, he provided me with insights from the greatest cultural works of the Western world. Louise, who is very sensitive, profound, calm, and wise, accepted me as I worked through my self-esteem issues. She was never shy to say, "I love you." But mainly, they both "just" listened.

Asking Questions

The purpose of any questioning you do is to help your friend clarify her thinking. She is in a predicament to which there are no right or wrong answers and no solutions. So don't try to use your problem-solving skills here. She doesn't need advice. She needs your attentive and continual presence and your occasional question.

Your questions can be a relief to her. "Thank heaven you asked me that!" she may feel. "At last I can unload these feelings to someone!"

Here are some general questions that may be useful to ask your friend:

> What do you feel like talking about?
> What are you worried about the most?
> What's going on in your head today?

Certain types of questions are helpful. Other types are not. Let's take a look at some examples.

> *Helpful*. Reflective questions like, "What do you think about the risks of chemotherapy?"
> *Not helpful*. Judgmental or evaluative questions like, "Don't you think chemotherapy is too risky?"
> *Helpful*. Open-ended questions like, "How do you feel about God these days?"

Not helpful. Closed-ended, "yes/no" questions like, "Do you still believe God loves you?"

Why? questions are perhaps the most unhelpful of all and generally should be avoided. To ask "Why?" is to give your friend the feeling that you are analyzing her, questioning her judgment, grilling her, and/or patronizing her.

All helpful questions invite reasoning and searching with an attitude of welcoming openness. Unhelpful questions close it off with a judgmental or know-it-all stance.

A tip: if you find yourself asking the unhelpful kind of questions, look inside your own heart. Are you really frightened? Often judgmental questions or statements flip out from our own fear. If we take time out and learn to deal with that fear, we can be more open and helpful to our friend.

Once you've asked a question, have the courage to wait for her answer. Cancer patients are dealing with a lot in their heads. Silence doesn't mean your friend doesn't want to answer. Rather, she is probably struggling to know where to begin, or how to put into words her own tumbled feelings. If you break in too quickly, you give the impression that you don't have the time or patience to wait for her reply, or that you weren't serious about asking in the first place.

Finally, a good questioner never corrects her friend's answer ("But before you said . . ."), rapid-fires a series of questions (this would be like a cross-examination), or finishes her friend's sentences for her. Verbal one-upmanship is found in destructive relationships, not in a caring friendship.

Don't assume this listening/questioning process is going to be a well-written drama. It is not going to flow beautifully. Instead, expect it to be jumpy and full of tangents. Different

personality types may well warrant slightly different question
ing approaches. If your friend is the quiet type you may need
to do more nudging. If she is impulsive you may want to help
her consider things more carefully.

Choose the right time and place for your listening/questioning
process. My friend Susan was a marvelous example of this.
Although she is an incredibly busy and successful professional,
Susan never gave me the impression she had to hurry me.
Instead, she allowed plenty of time for our conversations. She
knew that talking often occurs best over meals, and she wisely
chose restaurants that wouldn't rush us either. Plenty of healing
happened for me in the unpressured space Susan created.

Touching Your Friend

Stephanie Matthews Simonton is a clinical psychologist, founder of the Cancer Counseling and Research Center in Dallas,
and coauthor of the ground-breaking book *Getting Well Again*.
In her latest book, *The Healing Family*, she says, about the
incredible power of touch: "Nonverbal communication is sometimes more effective and moving . . . A person who is ill has
an increased need to be held and loved. In fact, it is sometimes
appropriate to compare a seriously ill patient to a small child
in terms of this need because both feel vulnerable and help-
less . . . Particularly for the patient who doesn't look attractive
or feel well, physical affection is one of the best ways to
communicate acceptance and love."

Touching your friend is one of the most healing things you
can do. When you touch her, she will be enabled to say, "I
have cancer—but I am not cancerous!" She will know that she
is not one of the "untouchables."

So touch. At the minimum, greet your friend with a touch,

and close the visit with a touch. Pat her head, squeeze her toe, grip her hand, give her a kiss on the cheek.

Now let me say that another way for emphasis. Pat his head, squeeze his toe, grip his hand, give him a kiss on the cheek. Notice the shift? Simonton comments, "Good friends can hold you, hug you, give a back rub, or simply hold your hand . . . This kind of physical affection is still easier for women friends in our society than for men; sadly, our cultural homophobia doesn't permit men to share their feelings or to hold one another as freely as it allows women to. But men, too, need this kind of nourishment—from other men, as well as from women." Hug your male friend, too.

Male or female, no two people are alike in what feels good to them. Don't assume you know what your friend will like. Ask, "What feels good?" "What do you like in the way of touch?" Some people will like to have their hair smoothed, some will enjoy getting a light back scratch, or a shoulder massage, some will delight in having their faces or hands stroked, some will find it soothing to have their feet washed.

If the opportunity presents itself and you are able, touch your friend during her difficult moments. The day the nurses arrived to remove my nasogastric tube, both my friends Polly and Rae happened to be there. They were given permission to remain in the room and were emotionally able to do so. They held my arms as the nurses pulled out foot and foot of tube. I felt so loved by my friends!

Not every patient will accept physical affection at first. Simonton notes, "When a patient rejects touch, it is important to respect his wishes." But don't give up after only one try. Instead, you might suggest less threatening approaches that still involve touching: offer to give a manicure or pedicure, to brush or shampoo your friend's hair or do her makeup, or to trim his beard or mustache, or give him a shave.

Touch became a powerful vehicle of comfort to me during my illness.

Three experiences gently and gradually prepared me to receive the touching I needed.

Long before my cancer struck, I was talking with my former minister, Rick. "How do I know God's will?" I was asking, in some sorrow. "Oh," he said, smiling. "You want some lap time with God." He might not have meant it literally, but I took it that way—that we humans can pass on God's love to one another through caring touch and holding.

Some time later, also before my diagnosis, my friend Polly and I had attended a hospice clinic. There we were educated about the soothing effects of stroking, massaging, and holding the seriously ill person. Polly and I practiced this therapeutic touch on each other, learning to massage shoulders, neck, back, and feet. This educational experience impressed me with the concept of the healing power of touch.

Finally, I had my own first-hand experience of the amazing power of therapeutic touch. It happened the night of my original surgery. My parents gave me the gift of a private nurse to be with me through that long night. And in my waking moments, as I swam up to consciousness through the haze of pain-killers, I realized the nurse was massaging my legs. It felt more than wonderful. It was the soothing reassurance of another human hand saying, "I am here. I am with you."

All of these things were stepping stones to prepare me to receive the two "touches" I still needed.

It was the midpoint of my chemotherapy and radiation treatment—the third long session. Instead of feeling any better, I felt worse and worse. I was not entirely sure how I could continue with the next two treatments. Sensing my exhaustion, Polly turned to me. "Would you like me to hold you?" she asked, referring to the "cradle-rock" technique we had learned in hospice. And I thought, "Thank God!" I was ready.

Gently pushing aside the six tubes that twined their way into my body, she climbed into that bed with me and circled me with her arms. As she held me, I experienced the emotional release I so desperately needed. I was able to cry.

Yes, there was the risk of what-would-people-think if they saw us. Anyone who had been trained in therapeutic touch would recognize the "cradle-rock," but others might misunderstand. Yes, there was the risk that I would take offense. But I bless Polly for taking those risks. The healing benefit to me was far greater than the risks of being misunderstood. When Polly held me, I got my "lap time with God." In the person of a member of his Body on earth, I do believe God held me that night.

Healing touch is no stranger to the Christian community. It is fully a New Testament concept. And it was not long before I was to experience that collective touch of hope and healing.

Donna, Rick's wife, first suggested it to me. "Amy, what would you think of a laying on of hands service?" she asked. (Note, by the way, that she *asked*. She didn't say, *"You should."* This is a perfect example of how friends can broaden the patient's options through a caring question.)

Because she was the one who asked, I was willing to be open to the possibility. After all, this was Donna, whom I knew and trusted. "Fine," I said. "I'm open."

I was disappointed to learn that Donna and Rick would be on vacation the Sunday I was able to travel the 45 miles back to my old church. But I gamely went ahead with it.

At the end of the regular service, most of the people were already out on the lawn before the curate asked me on the church step, "Do you want a laying on of hands? Rick said you might come."

When I said yes and he announced it, a dozen and a half people standing on the lawn put aside their brunch dates or whatever, turned around, and came back inside the sanctuary.

I was anointed with oil and invited up to the altar rail. Behind me, hands stretched out to rest on my head and touch my back and shoulders, and people prayed for me. I don't really remember what they said. I do remember that I prayed a prayer of thanksgiving.

I'm told I radiated a light that was overwhelming to people in that sanctuary. They say I was aglow. I know I was aglow with thanksgiving.

I can't say for sure what happened that day. But I know that I am alive today, eighteen months later. My success story is being celebrated by people of both camps—the oncology team and those who laid hands on me. It's really pointless to argue whether the healing I enjoy so far is a result of either medical or spiritual help. I believe it was both. The medical treatments helped my body fight the cancerous cells. But the laying on of hands—the healing touch—definitely enhanced my emotional and connecting needs and nurtured my spiritual self.

Praying for Your Friend
Prayer is a gift you can always give. It costs nothing and takes so little time—yet the results are tremendous! Sometimes I knew when I was being prayed for—I could feel the prayers. These prayers reminded me of coasting in a glider on the

thermal winds over the Mojave desert the summer before—an invisible, yet powerful, uplifting of my spirit and my energy.

Praying for your friend can take many different forms.

One of the ministers at Fourth Presbyterian Church, Deborah, came to pray for me the night before my surgery.

After my hospitalization I went to see my friend Carolyn, who on my arrival turned to Abigail, her four-year-old, and said, "Remember when we prayed for Amy last year?" I got a mental image of mother and child praying for me at bedtime. What a sweet scene. And what a tremendous impact!

My friend Pat told her mother about my illness. Her mother took my name to her women's Bible study and prayer group, and they put me on a prayer chain. It was wonderful to have people who didn't even know me praying for me!

I found great comfort also when I received a note from the St. Margaret's Guild of St. Mark's church: "You're on our prayer chain."

I was ministered to by the praise and prayer of others—when they probably didn't even know it. As I sat in the pew at Fourth Presbyterian and all the voices around me raised their song of praise in the Doxology, I found myself in a "faith womb"— loved and supported by their faith-full worship.

What should you pray for? Personally, I want people to pray not so much for my healing, but for my health. Pray for my holistic health—the "wellness" of my heart, soul, mind, and body. Pray also for my acceptance of my condition, and that I will have the courage to cope with the consequences of my treatment. In her autobiographical book *When Your Friend Is Dying,* cancer patient Betsy Burnham says, "[Acceptance] does not mean being happy about [the] illness. Acceptance is relaxing; some would describe it as finding peace."

I didn't want conditional prayer, either. Too often, "Heal her," means "our will be done," not "thy will be done." I'm asking for the courage, the confidence, and the comfort to *accept* God's plan for me—not to *change* his plan for me. I'm asking that I will be enabled to accept his love for me as he wishes to express that love.

I signed up for an experimental protocol—a type of chemotherapy that has yet to be completely tested—to make my public statement to God, family, and friends, "I want to live." And I find solace in the Twenty-third Psalm: "Thy rod and thy staff they comfort me." I am letting go of holding on to life for my own sake, and I trust wholly in the Shepherd's guidance and caretaking.

6
Helping Your Friend Make Death and Dying Decisions (If Asked)

Remember the day you first heard your friend's diagnosis? You held your breath in the beginning. You cheered, struggled, and fought right alongside your friend as she toughed out each battle. You hoped against hope as the battles got longer.

And now it may be time for the quiet realization.

Your friend may be not *just sick*.

It is possible she may die, soon, as a result of her cancer.

As she herself comes into this awareness, she may ask for your help in making her final decisions and in coming to her final acceptance.

Some people may go through this process earlier rather than later. When I was given my final prognosis, it was as if someone had pushed the fast-forward button on my videotape machine.

I couldn't help playing through the tape to the probable end of the scene.

This chapter will help you give your friend information she may need to make those final decisions. Once more, you can serve as a resource to your friend as she is faced with the many difficult dilemmas surrounding her dying.

Your support may make the difference between your friend's facing these issues at all—or leaving them unresolved. For her to procrastinate on these issues is to sap the energy she needs for acceptance, transition, and passage.

Unresolved decisions are also time-bombs that wreak havoc in the family when your friend does die. "What did she really want for her funeral?" the family must then ask. Or they may forever agonize, "Were we right in allowing her to die by signing the Do-not-resuscitate order?" If the patient has not made these decisions for herself, her spouse, children, or other family members may live with lasting guilt as they question whether they made the wrong judgment call.

Your support can also help your friend come to a place of acceptance. What is it to accept one's own death? It is to understand one's identity and one's belongingness. It is to come to a place of wholeness, completeness, and peace.

The decisions your dying friend must deal with involve faith and ethical issues in two areas: treatment decisions, and decisions surrounding her death.

Treatment Decisions

Modern medical science is still struggling to treat the whole person, not just the body. Sadly enough, many patient's rights are still overlooked in treatment decisions. You can serve as an advocate for your friend to see that her rights are protected in three areas: 1) informed consent, 2) shared decision-making, and 3) hospice care. Your question to the medical team and to the family should always be, "Is my friend being told the whole truth?"

Informed consent. Unfortunately, some members of the medical profession still find it easier to give information to a family member rather than directly to the patient herself. Sometimes family members themselves complicate the communication process. "If you tell her, I'll never forgive you," a spouse may vow, fearing the patient will give up if she learns the truth.

But every patient has a right to know the truth. The President's Commission for the Study of Ethical Problems in Medicine and Biomedical and Behavioral Research says that "informed consent" means your friend has a right to know:

—her current medical status, which includes the likely course of the disease if no treatment is pursued.

—a complete description of all possible treatments, including the risks and benefits of each.

—the physician's professional opinion as to what is the best course of action.

I was fortunate in having physicians who were frank with me. As I faced the decision about my treatment they told me, "The standard radiation treatment has less than a thirty-percent cure prognosis."

As I wrote earlier, I asked for further information. "Who in your experience has lived to the magic five-year mark with my type and spread of cancer?"

My doctor responded honestly, "No one."

This information helped me make my choice about treatment. I signed up for the experimental protocol, about which the oncology team gave me equally frank information. "The experimental chemotherapy protocol is just that—experimental. We have some promising indications, but no data as yet."

But too often such frankness isn't the scenario. In that case, consider going to bat for your friend. Find out who has the information she needs to know and help see that she gets it. It's her right. If your friend feels she is not being told the truth consider going to her doctor's office with her to get the facts. Talk over this possibility with your friend. She may be relieved to have your loving support there with her. You can also help your friend identify what questions she wants to ask the doctor and take notes to help her remember the doctor's answers.

Shared decision-making. "The patient is so sick and stressed that her opinion isn't valid. We will make the decision for her." Unfortunately, this thinking still permeates too many hospital corridors.

The patient can usually make decisions. She should be given a voice in them. After all, they are decisions about her life.

The President's Commission agrees with this. Reporting in their 1982 U.S. government publication, called *Making Healthcare Decisions,* the Commission recommended that "the patient and provider collaborate in a continuing process intended to make decisions that will advance the patient's interests both in health (and well-being generally) and in self-determination." This is shared decision-making at its ideal. No one should interfere with this basic right of a patient, including you.

As she pursues self-determination, your friend may have to make some hard choices. She may opt for experimental drugs. She might consider alternative therapies or nontraditional methods of treatment. Or she may opt to end treatment. "Family, friends, and caregivers may find it hard to accept, but the time may come when continuing to live is no longer a patient's top priority," states a 1984 U.S. Department of Heath and Human Services booklet entitled, "Advanced Cancer: Living each Day."

Hospice care. One important right your friend has as a patient is for hospice care. The concept of hospice is care, not cure. Hospice places the accent on concern for quality of life, not prolonging life. Hospice care stresses controlling pain and maximizing the patient's comfort, as well as caring for the patient's emotional and spiritual health. Hospice is concerned for the needs of family members as well as those of patients.

Hospice emphasizes the quality of the care approach more than the type of facility used. Hospices exist throughout the United States and Canada, some as free-standing hospices, some as hospices within a particular hospital, and some as at-home care arrangements within a community. You can find out more about hospices in your area by writing to the *National Hospice Organization,* 1901 North Fort Meyer Drive, Arlington, VA 22209 or calling 1(703) 243-5900.

Drawing up documents. Should your friend opt to end treatment, she will need to protect her intention to do so. In the event that she becomes, for instance, comatose, she needs to have some type of document stating her wishes and appropriate instructions, for example, her preference regarding Do Not Resuscitate Orders (DNR).

There are three such types of documents your friend can have drawn up.

—*The "living will."* This legal document states that the patient does not wish to be kept alive by artificial means or heroic measures. It's wise for your friend to place a copy of the living will in a safe deposit box, to inform medical personnel and a responsible party of its existence, and also to make sure her lawyer and/or one of her friends or family members has a key to the box.

A sample of a living will from *When Your Friend is Dying,* by Edward Dobihel, Jr. and Charles Stewart, is shown here. Copies are available from the *American Protestant Health Association,* 1701 E. Woodfield Road, Schaumburg, IL 60195. Slightly different forms are available from the *Catholic Health Association,* St. Louis, MO 63134, and from *Concern for Dying,* 250 West 57th St, New York, NY 10019.

A Living Will
Instructions for My Care
in the Event
of Terminal Illness

My faith affirms that life is a gift of God and that physical death is a part of life, the completed stage of a person's development. My faith assures me that even in death there is hope and the sustaining grace and love of God. Because of my belief, I wish this statement to stand as the testament of my wishes.

I, _____
request that I be fully informed as my death approaches. If possible, I wish to participate in decisions regarding my med-

ical treatment and the procedures that may be used to prolong my life. If there is no reasonable expectation of my recovery from physical or mental disability, I direct my physician and all medical personnel not to prolong my life by artificial or mechanical means. I direct that I receive pain and symptom control. However, this is not a request that direct intervention be taken to shorten my life.

This decision is made after consideration and reflection. I direct that all legal means be taken to support my choice. In the carrying out of my will as stated, I release all physicians and other health personnel, all institutions and their employees, and all members of my family from legal culpability and responsibility.

Signed _____

Date _____

Witnessed by _____

_____

(Sign and date in the presence of two witnesses.)

—*Advance directive to physician.* Unlike the generality of the living will, an advance directive to your friend's physician can give specific instructions relating to your friend's particular case. Such a document helps absolve the physician from liability and minimizes his or her fear of a malpractice suit.

—*Durable power of attorney for health care.* With this document, your friend authorizes someone she knows and trusts to make decisions for her in the event she is not able to make them for herself.

Self-deliverance. There is another very difficult ethical consideration your friend will wrestle with. That is the question of self-deliverance.

In his book, *The Last Thing We Talk About,* noted evangelical author and educator the late Joseph Bayly described one man's decision to choose self-deliverance. "A few years ago a friend of mine, a godly man who had responded with courage and acceptance to the burden of cancer for many months, was in the hospital, weak and dying. His doctor had told him and his wife that he could not live longer than a week or two. One Sunday night, after a beautiful final visit with his wife, alone after her departure, my friend pulled the needle that was sustaining his life from his arm, shut off the valve, rolled up the tube and went to sleep. The next day he died."

"Did he take his own life?" asks Bayly. "No, I believe not," he continues. "What he did was merely to remove the means by which the doctor could delay his death for a few days, prolonging the suffering of his wife, delaying his soul's flight to God."

I also thought about this subject—couldn't avoid it! After reading two books on the subject, I choose to have faith in God's timing (but the fact remains that I haven't really had to deal with this issue personally yet).

Each of these difficult ethical decisions can be seen from differing faith perspectives, and self-deliverance is no exception. There are those who would say that self-deliverance is not acceptable for a person of faith, since God's gift of life is sacred and should be fought for and prolonged at all costs.

And there are those of equally sound faith who would say that it is acceptable—that death is simply a part of life.

Whichever stance your friend finally takes, it is not up to you to challenge her. Your support is what she needs, and your respect for her choice. Even clergy and denominations are still struggling over these complex ethical questions. How much more the average layperson?

So, respect your friend's choice. Consider that, as writer Lisa Sowle Cahill says in an article in the journal *Second Opinion,* published by the Lutheran General Healthcare System, "There are few . . . concrete moral issues about which Scripture pronounces a single clear and definitive answer . . . This is particularly true in the moral evaluation of healthcare, because most of its present-day forms and possibilities were unknown to the communities that produced the Bible and early Christian literature."

As to the church's responsibility to support, nurture, and care for the terminally ill and those faced with these crushing decisions, Kenneth L. Vaux, Professor of Ethics and Medicine at the University of Illinois Medical Center writes in *Health and Medicine in the Reformed Tradition:* "Churches and synagogues (which first received the commission to stand by those in need) must reenter the health care system . . . [They] should develop congregation-based clinics . . . For the terminally ill, the churches could develop extensive ministries of preparation, home-care, and companionship."

Decisions Surrounding Death

From the ages of eight to fourteen, I swam backstroke in YMCA competitions. As anyone who has swum backstroke knows, you're always afraid of hitting the end of the pool hard—either with your head or your hand. So you "spot" the ceiling, looking for markers. You try to gauge how close you are to the end.

Taking care of the concrete details surrounding a cancer patient's own death is a lot like that. Setting her will in order, tidying up other personal and business papers, arranging for her funeral and burial—all these are markers. Dealing with them gives your friend a sense of approach and confidence that the end is within reach and only requires a few more strokes. It alleviates her fear of reaching the end of the lane unprepared. It frees her to swim the race to the finish and win.

Here are some of the markers you can help your friend spot.

Updating a will. Is your friend currently thinking the same way she was when she initially made her will? Have her relationships with people mentioned in the will changed? Might she now wish to make contributions to charitable causes such as a hospice or the *American Cancer Society?*

Bequeathing her body. For some people, this may be a ridiculous point. They have no wish to bequeath their bodies and that's that. For others, it may be a way to say, "Precisely because of its cancerous condition, my body could be useful to medical science." The choice is a very personal one.

For myself, the decision to donate my body involved some faith questions. When I came to the understanding that my body did not have to remain intact in order to be resurrected, I felt quite comfortable about bequeathing it.

In Illinois where I live, bequeathing one's body is a matter of signing the appropriate spot on the driver's license—in the presence of and with the signatures of two witnesses. I asked my friend Polly and her daughter Barbara to be my witnesses.

"I feel very uncomfortable doing this," Polly admitted to me. But she was able to overcome her own reluctance, honor my wishes, and sign.

Choosing a cemetery. My decision to bequeath my body to medical science meant that I did not need to choose a cemetery. Some people might want to have a marker of some sort erected as a comfort to the family even if they do bequeath their bodies.

If your friend will need cemetery arrangements, she will have to decide whether she will be buried in a local cemetery or the family plot. If the family plot, will she choose the matriarchal line or the patriarchal? Or, if she has a spouse, will she choose to be buried where he will be?

Giving direction for the funeral or memorial service. The funeral service may have more meaning for your friend's family than for her. But since most families want to take the last wishes of their loved one into consideration, your friend will want to let her wishes be known.

This is especially true in cases of differing faith convictions between your friend and her family. In an article in *The Anglican Digest,* writer Taschia Ann comments, "I am an Episcopalian, and I believe in Jesus' promise of life after death. My family does not. So I felt a real need to be sure that my death be taken care of correctly by the church and me. There is no doubt that the family will follow my wishes. But it is my responsibility to make those wishes clear."

Your supportive presence can be invaluable as your friend plans her funeral. I found I could not be alone as I began to write ideas for my memorial service. I needed to be in the companionship of loved ones.

So I went to Polly and Tom's showroom, and there, in the

emotional safety of their back room, a flood of memories swept over me. I had never attended a funeral of a close relative. However, I found myself reliving an event that had happened a year before.

On a beautiful summer day, I put my dog Precious in the car and drove back to where he and I used to live, for a farewell picnic. He was a five-dollar, from-the-pound dog, and I loved him dearly. After several happy years together, I found out that Precious had cancer—of a type that did not permit him to lie down. "He can't rest," the vet told me. "He's too sore." So I had made the hard decision to put Precious to sleep. Today was the day.

I chose for the picnic a spot where Precious used to walk morning, noon, and night, on the golf course tucked inbetween the woods and the creek. As I set up the picnic of his favorite "people" foods—salami and cheeses and chocolate chip cookies—he scampered off to renew his acquaintances with ducks, squirrels, and rabbits, then hurried back to sniff and inhale the goods.

After about an hour and a half I knew the picnic couldn't go on forever. I watched him run up that long fairway with his customary crooked gallop for the last time, ears flying, tail wagging. He clambered in the car and, as my copilot, stuck his head out of the window as we headed for the vet.

I held him as he was injected. I held him as he fell. I held him as he cooled down.

Then I walked out.

My first stop was a local florist, where I bought a rose. I proceeded immediately to St. Mark's, where I had worshipped for many years. The church was empty. I walked up the aisle to the railing and put the rose down. Then I prostrated myself, prayed for my dog, and cried for me. I thanked God that my dog had been part of my life. And sometime, I don't know, maybe fifteen minutes later, I got up and went back out to my car.

My next stop was a music store, where I bought a tape of the Canadian Brass playing Vivaldi. I returned to the old neighborhood and I rolled back the sunroof. I pealed those trumpets as loudly as I could as I crisscrossed every block Precious and I had walked on our evening walks.

And then I went home.

Alone.

He was a wonderful friend.

In my mind I had this replay as I sat there in Polly and Tom's office with my empty pad of paper. I realized that what I had done for Precious was what I wanted done for me. Then the writing of my own funeral just flowed. I made decisions, and I made them easily.

Notifying friends and loved ones. Your friend will need to decide who is to be notified at the event of her death. This notification can be as formal or as informal as she chooses. I recently received a formal death notice in the mail. Beautifully printed on elegant card stock, it read, "John C. Smith died of complications relating to cancer on December 10, 1986. A memorial fund has been set up in John's name for the *American Cancer Society,* New York, NY. Condolences may be sent to John's mother, Mrs. Henrietta Smith, at (address)."

To expedite this process, I have marked my address book. I've placed an asterisk next to each name I want notified by phone or mail, and a double asterisk next to those I want invited to my funeral.

Leaving a "legacy of love." *Legacy of Love: How to Make Life Easier for the Ones You leave Behind* is a workbook written by Elmo Petterle and published by Shelter Publications, Inc. It's one of the most useful ways I've seen to tidy up all the paperwork and pull together the decisions of will preparation and funeral arrangements with matters of life insurance, social security, medicare, veteran's benefits, pensions, IRA's, Keoghs, and other financial planning decisions and documents so that all trust and estate issues and survivor concerns can be more easily managed.

It's amazing the number of details that need to be managed as one faces death. It can be amusing, too, what will bother one person and not another. I myself had a fetish about cleaning out all my closets—and particularly about throwing away all my old shoes. I didn't want the church's social service group to have to do the give-away sorting for me. After all, some shoes cannot be reused!

I was also quite compulsive about getting my taxes in order. I didn't want to leave my parents with the hassle of trying to straighten that out.

Seeking and giving forgiveness. When they know they are going to die, many people discover that they want to both seek and give forgiveness. They feel a need to seal their friendship with God and with others. They want to make amends.

Don't be surprised if your friend leans on you for support as she faces this task. You might be inclined to discourage her from doing it because you know—and you're right—that she'll open old wounds and feel the hurt again. Yet she knows that she has a gift to give and it's worth giving. That gift is calling and saying, "I love you. I always have and I always will."

Walk with your friend through these death and dying decisions. Don't run ahead; don't lag behind. She will gain comfort from your presence.

What Awaits Your Friend After Death?

Not long before my cancer crisis, I was fortunate enough to tour the Holy Land with fellow worshipers and friends. During the trip, I bought one important memento. It's a silver statue of Caleb and Joshua hefting a huge bunch of grapes on a pole between them. That statue has come to be a visible reminder of my trust for the future. Yes, there is a Promised Land.

Most people sooner or later do grapple with this question, perhaps life's biggest: Is there life after death? For the cancer patient, that question is pressing.

For me, death is just a transition. It is a window to the world of God's everlasting life.

I anticipate and long to find that next "Aha!" place with God. I know it will top all those periods of wonder and awe I have ever experienced.

I look forward to it with the trust a child must have when he's birthed: not knowing, but trusting. It will be a crescendo— bigger and better. Each wave will lap up what's been before and bring a new wonder.

It will be like the eagerness to wake up Christmas morning, and the breathless waiting for everyone to gather around the Christmas tree.

It will be like the Grand Canyon—I will be bedazzled in total awe. I expect to take a step backwards, shield my eyes for a second and say, "I can't take it all in."

I know that then I will no longer question, "Am I lovable?" I will be in the presence of total acceptance—like being bathed in the water of the ocean. Like basking in the warmth of the sun and the perfume of the garden with all the splendor of its colors. And I will be a shape, a texture, a color, a fragrance, complementing the whole.

Heaven is the jigsaw puzzle where all the pieces fit—where what comes together is beyond the senses and requires a sixth sense to comprehend. It will be the notes we cannot hear here. I need music, dance, painting, and poetry to speak of such a place.

Yes, my Joshua and Caleb sculpture reminds me there is a heaven ahead. But there is a heaven here on earth as well. "He walks with me and he talks with me and he tells me I am his own." A cancer crisis can put your friend into a closer walk with God. And into the direct presence of the Almighty.

7
Being There
for Your Friend

Cancer is such a strange disease. Its relapses and remissions, recurrences and respites wash back and forth like the ebb and flow of the tide. Is the tide going out? Or is it coming in? Sometimes it's hard to tell. The course of the disease is not linear.

One half of all cancer patients will survive five years or more. Chances are that at some point your friend will leave the crisis stage of intense treatment, where she anticipates death. She will move into a stage of "remission"—of waiting to see what happens next. And it will be possible—and necessary—for her to reenter the world.

Reentry brings with it a whole new set of adjustments for your friend and calls for a whole new set of responses from you.

Survivorship

Because your friend has had cancer, she has moved into a whole new identity in the community. The cancer patient is now formally considered to be one of the "handicapped" by the Federal government's Rehabilitation Act of 1973. The average person thinks of the cancer patient as a cancer "victim."

Dr. Fitzhugh Mullan, himself a former cancer patient, advocates the use of the term "survivor" to give the cancer patient a more positive identity. Writing in a recent issue of the *New England Journal of Medicine,* Mullan says, "Survival begins at the point of diagnosis, because that is the time when patients are forced to confront their mortality and begin to make adjustments that will be part of their immediate and, to some extent, long-term future."

Mullan describes three "seasons of survival": the acute, the extended, and the permanent survival seasons.

The acute survival season is dominated by the cancer treatment. This is the crisis phase.

The extended survival season is dominated by fear of recurrence—"the punishing worry that the tumor, now in abeyance, will return to resume its perfidious work," says Mullan.

The permanent survival season, Mullan suggests, is "roughly equated with the phenomenon we call cure." Again, recall the statistics. Fifty percent of those diagnosed with cancer will survive to this point.

The first six chapters of this book have dealt with the acute survival season and teaching you how to help your friend through her crisis. But this chapter will deal with the extended survival season. It will teach you how to respond to your friend as she moves from her crisis orientation to her chronic orientation. Most cancer patients are in this extended survival season, which spans the first three to five (or more) years after the patient's diagnosis and treatment. It is in this extended survival season that your friend reenters the real world. As she does, she faces reentry issues in two areas: medical and social.

Medical issues. Recurrence and rehabilitation are the two biggest concerns your friend has, medically speaking.

In the fifteen months following my treatment, I encountered three separate health-related concerns. Each one brought on fears of recurrence.

My first scare came when six months after treatment I developed rectal bleeding. Immediately I feared the worst: metastasis of the cancer to the colon. But after undergoing many tests, I was relieved to find out that the bleeding was "only" due to radiation damage to my colon from the initial treatments.

A second scare came ten months after treatment, when I developed a cough and lost my voice. Fears of lung cancer set in, and again I underwent an extensive battery of tests. The tests turned up nothing physical—and my physician concluded that my voice loss was due to the stress I had put it under—a three-day speaking tour de force that had me jet-hopping to three major cities in as many days. I breathed a sigh of relief and slowed down my schedule.

My most recent scare came fifteen months after treatment—vaginal bleeding. This one really threw me because it seemed linked to the original site of the cancer. But again, tests showed that the bleeding was actually from the bladder—still one more result of radiation damage.

I tell these stories to illustrate to you how each physical symptom, be it "small" or large, becomes magnified to the cancer patient. It's no longer a matter of a simple cough, fever, or runny nose. Each time her thought is, "Is it the cancer?"

Rehabilitation is another concern for your friend. I was very fortunate not to have any visible signs of being a treated cancer patient. Some people, however, must cope with reentry into society minus an arm or a leg, or with visible scarring. The adjustment can be tough.

However, I was impacted emotionally, and had to cope with readjustment to life given the new realities of my situation.

Social issues. Social concerns your friend will face include community acceptance, insurance discrimination, and barriers to employment. Again, let me share from my experiences to illustrate these points.

My particular form of cancer raised for me serious questions about my acceptability. I walked around with the scarlet letter feeling, because if my friends were to do what I had suggested and get the *American Cancer Society* printout on cervical cancer, they would read some things that might cause them to wonder about me. Cervical cancer, the printout would say, usually happens to women of lower socioeconomic class who have engaged in early sexual activity and with multiple partners.

I did not fit this profile. Yet I felt my morality was labeled by my cancer label. (As a matter of fact, I reacted so strongly to this label when I first heard it that I argued with the doctor. "No," I insisted. "You must have it wrong. I can't possibly have cervical cancer—I don't fit the profile. It must be uterine cancer. That's the profile—that's me!")

Eventually, I came to realize that just as there are people who get lung cancer who never smoked a day in their lives, so there are people who get cervical cancer who don't fit the statistical profile.

Dating also became a problem for me. In the beginning, I

was much too blunt. When asked the typical, "Hi! Tell me about yourself and what you've been doing for the last six months," I would tell them. And that would be the end of that. They'd never call back or ask for a second date. Finally my friend Rae took me aside. "I know you've got this thing for being honest," she said. "But I don't think it's in your best interest to be that candid!"

She may be right—but when I look at my situation very realistically, I still have to ask, "Given my prognosis, who would want to get involved with me?"

Insurance discrimination is a very real reentry problem for cancer patients. Although there are many movements right now to get insurance for us, the problem still remains.

I was fortunate in having great medical coverage. But I didn't have disability insurance or life insurance, which I will always regret. A couple of months after my treatment, when I received a direct mail ad to buy some life insurance, I decided to test the waters. And sure enough, I was turned down.

A humorous sideline to that story is that I did get a follow-up mailer from that same company—in which they tried to sell me stocks! I really had to laugh—they knew they wouldn't get their money out of me life-insurance-wise; but they sure might stock-wise. This time, I turned *them* down.

Barriers to employment for cancer patients are also a real problem. As reported in a 1987 *Crain's Chicago Business* article headlined, "Cancer on the Job: Recovery doesn't blunt discrimination," an *American Cancer Society* study found these disturbing facts. One out of four recovered patients has experienced work-related discrimination in some form because of his or her medical history. This discrimination takes the forms of being ostracized by coworkers, being demoted or not promoted, being fired, or failing to be hired because some managers erroneously believe that in all cases a company's insurance rates automatically rise if someone on the payroll turns in large medical bills.

The problem is slightly worse for blue-collar workers. A study of 211 cancer patients, funded by the California division of the *American Cancer Society* and reported in *USA Today*, found that over five years, fifty percent of the white collar workers and eighty-four percent of the blue collar workers suffered either outright discrimination or other problems because of their cancer.

Since I am self-employed, cancer affects my career slightly differently. I can at least promote myself and give myself a new title. But I'm not on a payroll! Each time I take on a new client, I must ask myself how much to tell. No, I am not required to submit a medical history. But what is ethical?

That Humpty Dumpty Feeling

The main thing for you to grasp is that your friend will never be the same again. As Dr. Mullan states, "Whatever our wishes, the person who has come through a cancer experience is indelibly affected by it. For better or for worse, physically and emotionally, the experience leaves an impression."

It's much like the Humpty Dumpty fairy tale. No matter how much they tried, "all the king's horses and all the king's men couldn't put Humpty together again." There's no such thing as "as good as new." Your friend's point of view is forever altered.

What may seem like just an ordinary occurrence can have larger effects. Let me illustrate with five normal routines from my recent past.

—I turned on the television one night—and there was a program about C.S. Lewis's dealing with his wife Joy's terminal phase of cancer. I learned that he did in fact marry her when she had cancer. Although I know this is a rare occurrence, sitting there in my apartment alone, I lamented that I didn't have anyone. "God," I said, "why don't you give me a C.S. Lewis?"

—I went to a movie with a friend. We both felt like we needed a good laugh; this movie seemed likely to afford that, though neither of us had read the reviews. But in the opening scene, the protagonist had an out-of-body experience and went into frantic ravings about cancer killing everyone. Our nice night out together had turned into an uncomfortable one.

—My parents asked me if I would get a portrait made. This was a perfectly normal request—but under the circumstances I couldn't help thinking about the reasons. Why did they want the portrait? To remember me by. As I chose my outfit and did my makeup for the sitting, I became almost obsessed with the idea: "I am dressing to be remembered forever."

—During a seminar presentation I was doing for some clients, I developed a cough. But because I was afraid they'd think it was another symptom of my cancer, I didn't even want to clear my throat! I had visions of them taking me aside and saying, "We'll pay you for a full day, but you don't need to continue beyond the afternoon coffee break, thank you."

—I attended the fundraiser of my local hospice. It was the same fundraiser I had attended the year before. Then, I was simply attending out of sincere but generalized support. This year, I had a vested interest in raising those funds. I wanted this hospice to be in good shape should I need it!

These are just a few of the ways life gets turned on its head for the cancer patient. Any of these "simple" events can suddenly become the occasion of momentary emotional "cardiac arrest" for your friend.

You can help her best by continuing to be there.

Being There

In *USA Today,* Dr. Sarah Splaver, a survivor of breast cancer and founder of the support group "CHUMS," writes, "Cancer patients speak of two losses. "[Number] one is the loss of their friends."

Simply, we cancer patients fear the loss of our friends.

But a true friend never gives up. Robert L. Veninga, whose close friend died of a long illness, writes in his book *A Gift of Hope,* "Stripped of all its other definitions, a friendship affirms that we will not be abandoned."

The extended season of survival gives you a chance to show your true friendship by not abandoning your friend. Simply put, by being there.

"Being there" means just that. You can't keep sending flowers forever. There's not necessarily any more crisis discussion.

What you can offer now is hospitality—a place and a space to be there with your friend. Speaking of our task as lay people to be healers, Henri J. M. Nouwen writes the following in his book *Reaching Out:* "As healers we have to offer safe boundaries within which the often painful past can be revealed and the search for a new life can find a start . . . Healing is the humble but also very demanding task of creating and offering a friendly empty space where strangers can reflect on their pain and suffering without fear, and find the confidence that makes them look for new ways right in the center of their confusion."

You see, your friend has likely made a crossover. She has met the challenge of figuring out how to die well. But death has not yet arrived—and may not for quite some time. She still has a few strokes left to swim in her backstroke race. So she now has a new challenge: figuring out how to live. How to live within her new limits. How to live within her new labels. How to live.

As I went through my "how do I live now?" phase, I first found I needed some R and R. "I'm coming out to live again, and I need my friends to just keep me company," was my feeling. My friends Mary and Andrew did exactly that. They opened their apartment in New York to me and we had some delightful weekends in the Big Apple. A leisurely Saturday brunch, an afternoon stroll in Soho, an evening of jazz at the Blue Note. On the way home we'd buy the *New York Times* and stop at *David's cookies,* then read the paper and munch till the wee hours. We didn't talk cancer.

Anytime I'm in the blues, I need new beginnings. As I began to walk out of my post-treatment blues, my friend Shirley became very important to me. Her children, Brad, five, and Kerry, three, were new beginnings to me at a time when I was trying to get out of endings.

Another friend, also named Mary, offered me a great gift when she moved to Washington D.C. "I had you in mind when I picked out our home," she told me. "There's space for you in Washington should you need it."

Linda and Peter sent faithful cards for all those normal everyday occasions—Christmas, birthday, Valentine's. They hadn't "crossed me off" their list.

Barbara sent a "no occasion" card—just to let me know she was thinking of me. The card had "rainbow seeds" in it—popcorn-sized pieces of bright velour. "Plant these and they'll grow a rainbow," it said.

Soon, it became time to resume work: I felt stronger. But should I continue on with my consulting business? What should I do? I found myself retooling a longer-term game plan.

Any time one retools her game plan, she needs resources. In this juncture of wanting to have a new beginning but being without resources, parents and families can prove they are friends. My parents did just that. In the theater, donors who fund the production of a show are fondly referred to as "angels." My parents became my "angels" by offering to subsidize me to do whatever I wanted—whether it was to volunteer for cancer causes, or whatever. They offered to underwrite my "show." Though I did decide to continue on with my consulting business, it was comforting to know I had options for a backup position.

Potential Traps in "Being There"

As you hang in there with your friend, watch out for these potential pitfalls.

Lack of reciprocal reward. What you gave your friend may likely have exceeded what you got back during her crisis phase. This imbalance of giving can't go on forever. Sooner or later, your friend is going to start to feel guilty if the relationship is so one-way.

You need to begin sharing your own life concerns with your

friend again. Caring is done through sharing. Just because your friend has cancer doesn't mean she has lost her caring skills. Cancer hasn't stripped her of the stripes of friendship.

Polly and I went through this transition in our friendship. She wanted to keep being stoic for me so I could lean on her. That had been appropriate during the acute phase of my illness. But now, in the extended phase, what I wanted was for her to be vulnerable with me again. I needed to be needed. Fortunately, we were able to express these feelings to each other, and regain a balance of reciprocity. When it ceases to be reciprocal, a friendship is dead.

Lack of honesty. This is a related point, and it has to do with our tendency to tender-toes around the person who has had cancer. We are tempted to withhold information that we fear will be painful. But this is nothing more than lack of honesty, and it is very damaging.

For instance, I did not find out that my father's best friend had died from cancer until some months later. I suspect that my father had been concerned about telling me. When I did find out, I was sad, both because I hadn't been able to share his grief, and also because my illness had been the cause of a strain in communication.

Polly also withheld from me news of the cancer-related death of an instructor friend of hers. Of course in time I found out. Then there is that double barrier to overcome. "Why didn't you tell me?"

Obsession to always ask about the cancer. As time goes on, her cancer is no longer the headline story in your friend's life. Other banners lead the day. So when you ask her, "How are you?" don't expect always to hear more on the cancer story. Maybe the highlight of today is her terrific golf game. Let it be. Let her be doing great!

As you help your friend through her cancer crisis, take heart in remembering that each friend fills a specific niche in the Cosmic Care Plan. And maybe you'll discover, as I have, the truth of what C.S. Lewis wrote in *The Four Loves:* "For a Christian, there are, strictly speaking, no chances. A secret Master of the Ceremonies has been at work. Christ, who said to the disciples, 'Ye have not chosen me, but I have chosen you' can truly say to every group of Christian friends, 'You have not chosen one another, but I have chosen you for one another.' " God chooses our friends. And you are a very needed and special one.

Postscript

People often ask me these days how I'm doing. I reply, "I'm feeling healthy, wealthy, and wise!"

I'm healthy in the sense that I have tremendous peace and joy—a strong emotional and spiritual health.

And although I don't have a surplus in the bank, I have an abundance of love, care, and concern from my parents and friends—a true measure of wealth.

I'm wiser, too. I've learned so many things from my cancer experience! The following are only a few.

An Answer to the "Why?"
As I have written, when I got my "no one has lived" answer

from my doctor, I struggled with the huge question of "Why?" Was my cancer punishment? Did I do something terrible to deserve it? As I've gone through the crisis of cancer, I've begun to experience some healing answers to the "Why?" One incident in particular stands out.

It was right after my last week in the hospital. In preparation for a business trip, I decided to take all my good shoes in to the shoemaker and have them reheeled. I picked the shoes up at the appointed time, but when I got home, I discovered that none of them were fixed!

So I took all the shoes back and politely explained to the shoemaker what had happened.

But he started yelling and throwing a real fit! "You're trying to take me!" he screamed. "Those shoes were never in this shop!" I was absolutely bewildered, and left with the shoes unheeled.

Plainly, I did not deserve this kind of treatment. It was unjust and uncalled for. But it had happened.

The moral of this incident was so clear that I finally saw the same lesson in regard to my cancer. My cancer was not punishment. My cancer simply happened.

Rev. Russell Burck, a chaplain-supervisor at Rush-Presbyterian St. Luke's Medical Center, wrote a paper about this shift of thinking in 1981: "Thus our experience teaches us that such illness is not fairly distributed, and that we have to change our beliefs about the fairness of life."

This is one of my greatest learnings out of my cancer experience, best expressed by the cliché, "I never promised you a rose garden." I no longer take personal tragedies as God's punishment. I have a much stronger emotional health in knowing that what happens is not a measure of my worth.

The Upside of Cancer

Most cancer patients share a very wonderful perspective that cancer is not only a life-changing event, but a life-enriching one.

Betty Rollins, a breast cancer patient and author of the book, *First You Cry,* wrote the following in the *New York Times* in 1980, five years after her mastectomy: "Cancer enriched my life, made me wiser, made me happier. I am glad I had it." To which I can say a hearty "Amen," and also echo Betty Rollins when she says, "I was so struck by this apparent change in me—that the damage to my body had indeed done wonders for my head."

Ms. Rollins continues, "Cancer made me less worried about what people think of me both professionally and socially." As my learning goes on, I especially hope I grow to this stage, too.

Enjoying Today—Without Guilt

Betty Rollins also has something to say about the freedom to enjoy today. She writes, "I sop up pleasure where and when I can. Sometimes, at the risk of professional advancement, and sometimes at the risk of bankruptcy!"

My cancer has given my Protestant work ethic a jolt. I had always thought, "Work hard today for tomorrow's play." Now I am beginning to see with Ms. Rollins that I can enjoy hard— because I have today.

I also literally believe the message of Matthew 6:31: "Do not start worrying: 'Where will my food come from? or my drink? or my clothes?' Your Father in heaven knows that you need all these things. Instead, give first place to his Kingdom and to what he requires, and he will provide you with all these other things."

97

Tomorrow really will take care of itself. So enjoy today!

A Reason for Living

"A reason must be found for living with the limitations of illness or the [patient] will not," writes Sandra L. Grantstrom (R.N., M.S.N., D.Min.) in a recent study in *Topics in Clinical Nursing*. "In this quest," she continues, "all human beings must have something to believe in, something to hope for, and someone to love and return their love."

Finding this kind of meaning for my illness was a puzzle. But then I rediscovered a new meaning for the following poem which I had tucked away in my Bible. At the time my father gave it to me a few years ago, I couldn't relate to it and didn't know what it was for. Now it provides a framework for my cancer.

The Monument

God
before He sent His children to earth
gave each one of them
a very carefully selected package
of problems.

These,
he promised, smiling,
are yours alone. No one else
may have the blessings
these problems will bring you,
and only you
have the special talents and abilities

that will be needed
to make these problems
your servants.

Now go down to your birth
and to your forgetfulness.
Know that I love you beyond measure.
These problems that I give you
are a symbol of that love.
The monument you make of your life
will be a symbol of your love for Me.

Your father

—Anonymous

I have found tremendous satisfaction in writing this book. And as a result of what I've learned in the process, I've been asked to speak to professional associations, community organizations, and church groups about my cancer experience. I am in a position of service—and it's my problems that have enabled me! "Make these problems your servants." Had I not had my cancer, I wouldn't be doing these things I am getting so much pleasure out of!

My best wisdom is a profound appreciation of two pieces of Scripture. John 3:16, which so many of us know and love so well, says, "For God so loved the world that he gave his only begotten Son, that whosoever believeth in him should not perish, but have everlasting life" (John 3:16, KJV). Cancer can, and probably will, kill my cells and tissues, but it can never overcome God's promise of everlasting life.

And Philippians 4:13—"I can do all things through Christ who strengthens me." Not only can I cope with my broken parts, I can also accept the line in the Lord's Prayer: "Thy will be done."

I knew I had reached this acceptance of God's will one day as I was driving down a country road. A tree caught my attention. It was a beautiful pine with lush spreading boughs. Or it would have been—but all the branches had been sheared away on one side to allow the telephone wire to pass.

I am that tree. Because God had other plans for me, I was pared away here and there to let loving messages come through me to others.

As you read and share the message of this book, I pray that all the love I have felt and feel will pass through me to bless, enrich, and nurture you. And your friend.

With all my love,
Amy

Information Centers

Organizations:

The *American Cancer Society* (a private nonprofit organization)
1 (800) ACS–2345

The *Cancer Information Service* (coordinated by the National Cancer Institute, part of the U.S. Department of Health and Human Services)
1 (800) 4–CANCER

Seminars or Programs:

"I Can Cope" (educational seminars co-sponsored by the *American Cancer Society* and local hospitals)
90 Park Avenue
New York, NY 10016
1 (800) ACS–2345;
(212) 736–3030

Make Today Count
(a nonprofit national support
group for the terminally ill)
P.O. Box 222
Osage Beach, MO 65065
(314) 348–1619

CanSurmount
(American Cancer Society
one-on-one visitor program
where surviving cancer patients become volunteers to
help others deal with cancer)
90 Park Avenue
New York, NY 10016
1 (800) ACS–2345;
(212) 736–3030

International Association of
Laryngectomees (IAL)
(American Cancer Society
visitor program, site specific)
90 Park Avenue
New York, NY 10016
1 (800) ACS–2345;
(212) 736–3030

United Ostomy Association
(UAC)
(American Cancer Society
visitor program, site specific)
2001 W. Beverly Blvd.
Los Angeles, CA 90057
1 (800) ACS–2345;
(213) 413–5510

Reach to Recovery
(American Cancer Society
visitor program for breast
cancer patients, site specific)
90 Park Avenue
New York, NY 10016
1 (800) ACS–2345;
(212) 736–3030

Hospices:
The *National Hospice*
Organization
1901 N. Fort Meyer Drive
Suite 902
Arlington, VA 22209
(703) 243–5900

Making a Living Will:
Concern for Dying
250 West 57th Street
New York, NY 10019
(212) 246–6962

American Protestant Health
Association
1701 E. Woodfield Road
Schaumburg, IL 60195
(312) 843–2701

The Catholic Health
Association
4455 Woodson Road
St. Louis, MO 63134
(314) 427–2500

Suggested Literature:
Coping
P.O. Box 54693
Boulder, CO 80322
1 (800) 525–0643

"Listen with Your Heart: Talking with the Cancer Patient" (free pamphlet)
American Cancer Society
90 Park Avenue
New York, NY 10016
1 (800) ACS–2345;
(212) 736–3030

"Taking Time"
"Chemotherapy and You"
"Radiation Therapy and You"
(free pamphlets)
National Cancer Institute
U.S. Department of Health
and Human Services
1 (800) 4–CANCER

Bibliography

———. *1986 Cancer Facts and Figures*. New York: American Cancer Society, Inc., 1986.

———. *Coping with Cancer*. Washington, D.C.: U.S. Department of Health and Human Services, 1980.

Ann, Taschia. "A Goal for the Dying; Care of the Living" in *The Anglican Digest*, Advent 1986.

Bayly, Joseph. *The Last Thing We Talk About*. Elgin, IL: David C. Cook Publishing Company, 1973.

Burck, Rev. Russell, Ph.D. "Faith and Illness: Spiritual Resources for When We Are Ill," an unpublished paper, 1981.

Burnham, Betsy. *When Your Friend is Dying*. Grand Rapids, MI: Zondervan Publishing House, 1982.

Cahill, Lisa Sowle. "Ethical Issues in Medicine" from *Second*

Opinion: Health, Faith, and Ethics, Vol. 2. Park Ridge, IL: Park Ridge Center and Lutheran General Health Care System, 1986.

Connelly, Susan S. "Helping Patients Cope: The Role of the Patient Visitor in Cancer Care" in *The Journal of MAG,* Vol. 73, December 1984.

Cousins, Norman. *Anatomy of an Illness.* New York: Bantam Books, 1981.

Dobihal, Edward F., Jr. and Charles William Stewart. *When A Friend Is Dying.* Nashville: Abingdon Press, 1984.

Drakeford, John W. *The Awesome Power of the Listening Heart.* Grand Rapids, MI: Zondervan Publishing House, 1982.

Drimmer, Frederick, editor. *A Friend Is Someone Special.* Norwalk, CT: C.R. Gibson Company, 1975.

Farmer, Frances. *Will There Really Be a Morning?* New York: Putnam Publishing, n.d.

Fine, Judylaine. *Afraid to Ask.* New York: Lothrop, Lee and Shepard Books, 1984, 1986.

Fiore, Neil. *The Road Back to Health.* New York: Bantam Books, 1984.

Grantstrom, Sandra L. "Spiritual Nursing Care for Oncology Patients" in *Topics in Clinical Nursing,* April 1985.

Hansel, Tim. *You Gotta Keep Dancin'.* Elgin, IL: David C. Cook Publishing Company, 1985.

Hodge, James R., M.D. "Cancer Patients Need Help Coping with Fears, Changes" in *The Journal of Occupational Health and Safety,* April 1984.

Humphry, Derek. *Let Me Die Before I Wake.* Los Angeles, CA: The Hemlock Society, 1984.

Ireland, Jill. *Life Wish.* Boston: Little, Brown and Company, 1987.

Kushner, Harold S. *When Bad Things Happen to Good People.* New York: Schocken Books, An Avon Paperback, 1981.

Levenson, Dr. Frederick B. *The Anti-Cancer Marriage.* Briarcliffe Manor, NY: Stein and Day Publishers, 1987.

Lewis, C.S. *The Four Loves.* New York: Harcourt, Brace and World, 1960.

Marty, Martin E. *Friendship.* Allen, TX: Argus Communications, 1980.

Matthews-Simonton, Stephanie. *The Healing Family.* New York: Bantam Books, 1984.

Morra, Marion and Eve Potts. *Choices: Realistic Alternatives in Cancer Treatment.* New York: Avon Books, 1980, 1987.

Mullen, Dr. Fitzhugh. "Seasons of Survival: Reflections of a Physician with Cancer" in *New England Journal of Medicine,* Vol. 313, July 25, 1985, pp. 270–73.

National Cancer Institute. *Advanced Cancer: Living Each Day.* Washington, D.C.: U.S. Department of Health and Human Services, June 1984.

Nouwen, Henri J.M. *Reaching Out.* New York: Doubleday, 1975.

Ogilvie, Lloyd J. *Why Not?: Accept Christ's Healing and Wholeness.* Old Tappan, NJ: Fleming H. Revell Company, 1985.

Pesmen, Sandra. "Cancer on the Job: Recovery doesn't blunt discrimination" in *Crain's Chicago Business,* January 19, 1987.

Petterle, Elmo A. *Legacy of Love: A Workbook.* Bolinas, CA: Shelter Publications, 1986.

Pogrebin, Letty Cottin. *Among Friends.* New York: McGraw-Hill, 1987.

The President's Commission for the Study of Ethical Problems in Medicine and Biomedical and Behavioral Research. *De-*

ciding to Forego Life-Sustaining Treatment. Washington, D.C.: 1983.

The President's Commission for the Study of Ethical Problems in Medicine and Biomedical and Behavioral Research. *Making Healthcare Decisions*. Washington, D.C.: 1982.

Reeve, Pamela. *Faith Is*. Portland, OR: Multnomah Press, 1970.

Rollins, Betty. "The Best Years of My Life," the epilogue in *First, You Cry.*, New York: Harper and Row, 1980.

Rollins, Betty. *Last Wish*. New York: Simon and Schuster and Linden Press, 1985.

Schaffer, Ulrich. *Growing Into the Blue*. San Francisco: Harper and Row Publishers, 1984.

Sharp, Deborah. "Fighting Disease—and Discrimination" in *USA Today*, August 14, 1985.

Sibley, Brian, *C.S. Lewis: Through the Shadowlands*. Old Tappan, NJ: Fleming H. Revell Company, 1985.

Siebel, Machelle, M.D. et al. "Sexual Function after Surgical and Radiation Therapy for Cervical Carcinoma" in *Southern Medical Journal*, Vol. 75, No. 10, October 1982.

Simonton, O. Carl and Stephanie Matthews-Simonton. *Getting Well Again*. New York: Bantam Books, 1978.

Spingarn, Natalie Davis. *Hanging In There: Living Well on Borrowed Time*. Briarcliffe Manor, NY: Stein and Day Publishers, 1982.

Vaux, Kenneth L. *Health and Medicine in the Reformed Tradition*. New York: Crossroad Publishing Company, 1984.

Veninga, Robert L. *A Gift of Hope*. New York: Ballantine Books, 1985.

Welter, Paul. "When Your Friend Needs You" from *How to*

Help a Friend. Wheaton, IL: Tyndale House Publishers, 1978.

Youngner, Stuart J. "Do-Not-Resuscitate Orders: No Longer Secret, But Still a Problem" in *The Hastings Center Report*, Vol. 17, No. 1, February 1987.

Index

God's cosmic care, 35
Grace, 42
Guilt, 6, 32
Healing heart, 54
Heaven, 82
Hematologist, 19
Hodgkin's disease, 22
Honesty, 93
Hospice, 51, 71
Hospital, 39, 44
"I Can Cope" seminar, 50, 101
Informed consent, 69
Insurance, 87
Ireland, Jill, 55
Keller, Helen, 53
Kübler-Ross, Elizabeth, 31
Laughter, 43
Leukemia, 21-23
Liposarcoma, 23
Listening, 54
Living will, 71-73
Loss of control, 10
Lung cancer, 21-22
Lymphoma, 21, 23
"Make Today Count," 50, 102
Making Healthcare Decisions, 70
Malignant, 19
Marty, Martin, 54
Melanoma, 1, 20-22
Memorial service, 77
Metastasis, 17, 20, 23, 28
"The Monument," 98-99
Morra, Marion and Eve Potts, 3
Music, 40
Mutilation, 10
Myelomas, 23
Myosarcoma, 23
National Cancer Institute, 26, 102
National Hospice Association, 71
"Nest and tuck," 37

Ogilvie, Lloyd J., 4
Oncologist, 19, 28
Oncology, 19
Osteosarcoma, 23
"Ostomy Club," 50
Pogrebin, Letty Cottin, 6
Prayer, 63
Prognosis, 23-24
Radiation, 24, 28-29
Recurrence, 26-27, 85
Rehabilitation, 85-86
Remission, 83
Sarcomas, 22-23
Schuller, Robert, 30
Scripture, 42, 99
"Seasons of Survival," 84
Self-deliverance, 74-75
Seven warning signals, 18-19
Shock, 31
Simonton, O. Carl and Stephanie
Matthews-Simonton, 59
Site, 20-24
Skin cancer, 20-22
"Spirit and Breath," 50
Staging, 23
Suicide, 74
Surgery, 24, 28
Survival rates, 22
Survivorship, 84
Symptoms, 18-19
"Thy will be done," 65
Touch, 59-63
Toxic energy, 55
Trends in Survival, 22
Types of treatment, 24-26
U.S. Department of Health and
Human Services, 10
Upside of cancer, 97
Why me?", 53, 95-100
Will, 71-73, 76